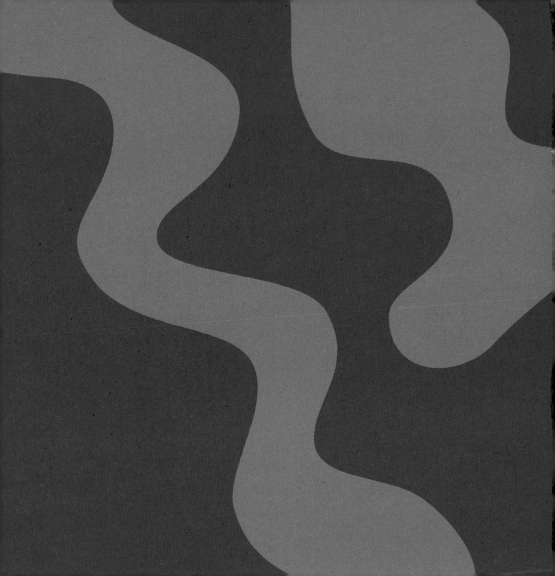

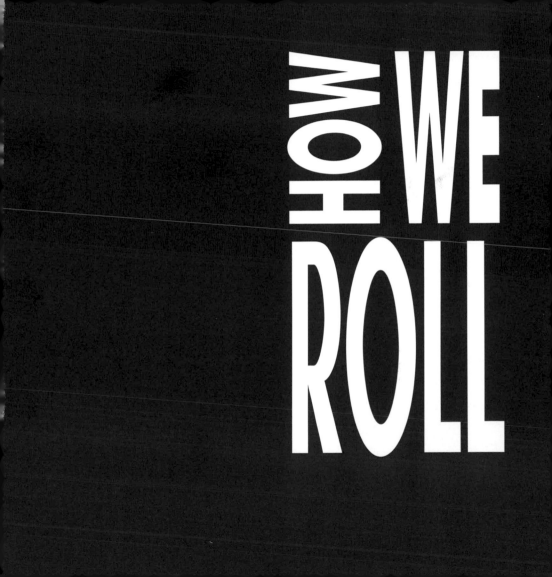

HOW WE ROLL

The Art and Culture of
JOINTS
BLUNTS
AND SPLIFFS

HOW WE ROLL

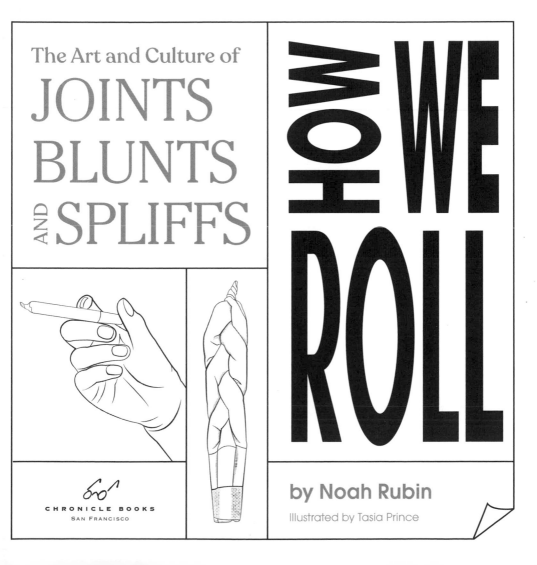

CHRONICLE BOOKS
SAN FRANCISCO

by Noah Rubin
Illustrated by Tasia Prince

Library of Congress
Cataloging-in-Publication Data available.
ISBN 978-1-7972-1293-7

Manufactured in India.

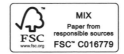

10 9 8 7 6 5 4 3 2

Chronicle Books LLC
680 Second Street
San Francisco, CA 94107

www.chroniclebooks.com

The information provided in this book is for educational purposes only. Please check with your local, state, and federal laws regarding consumption, possession, and cultivation of cannabis.

Tobacco use can be harmful to your health. Stay informed and do what's right for you. Neither the author nor the publisher received any payment or other consideration for the descriptions of tobacco products in this book.

Next to making a proper omelette or wiping your own ass, rolling a joint is an essential life skill for any self-respecting member of society.

- Anthony Bourdain

INTRODUCTION

It was the beginning of 2001, and I was living in southwest China near the border of Burma and Vietnam. The province is called Yunnan, and it was a needed change of scenery for me as I had just come from big city Beijing where I had lived for several months trying to learn Mandarin and desperately searching for any familiar fragment of the New York City lifestyle I had left behind, especially weed.

Besides traffic, pollution, and an occasional close call with a passerby's projectile wad of phlegm, the fact that weed was in very short supply in Beijing made me feel particularly far from home. When I did find a savory bit of cannabis it was always hash that had been trafficked in from the Xinjiang province near Afghanistan. To obtain this hash meant journeying to a hidden hutong alleyway that was also a de facto shooting gallery for many of the city's heroin users. Yunnan welcomed me with clean air and abundant natural beauty, but even more important was the discovery that I might be able to get my hands on some actual bud without an alleyway excursion.

"How much should I try to get?" my friend asked me excitedly after reporting that he had been approached by a smiling elderly farmer woman on the street holding a picture of plump nugs. "As much as you can, I guess." I responded with excitement, already visualizing the nostalgic and familiar joint I would roll after months of smoking nothing but pseudo–satisfying Xinjiang hash spliffs.

Little did I know what my response would summon because later that day when I caught up with my friend, he held a huge bag in his hands that looked a lot more like something from my late-fall childhood leaf-raking sessions in New England than the little baggies of weed I was used to buying in New York. "What's in there?" I naively asked. "It's the stuff," he replied. I couldn't believe my eyes. I had never seen so much weed in my life.

We immediately brought the sack back to our room and poured out the contents on a table. The quality was far from anything you could call high grade, but for whatever it may have lacked in potency it more than made up for in volume. Tackling this mountain of nugs would be no small task, so we enrolled a few friends who gladly joined us around the table as we began rolling joints. We couldn't roll fast enough, and as we lit up our joints, we'd take a few contemplative puffs and pass to the left. Our teamwork meant that as soon as we offered our joint to the person next to us, we were already receiving another joint through a halo of smoke from our right. The room quickly filled with a cloud of cannabis and as we approached an hour of nonstop rotation, our weedy cyclone summoned dreams of dumplings, another itch that would soon need to be scratched.

This book is about rolling joints, blunts, and spliffs, but it is also about the many unexpected possibilities that can emerge from this seemingly simple act. Writing and researching classic elevated rolls like the cross, the tulip, and the braid, led me to friends in the Caribbean who introduced me to the Trinidadian Roll On—a spliff unlike anything I had ever encountered. Similarly, as I prepared my description of numerous blunt rolling techniques, from classic cigar wraps to Fronto Leaf, I also wanted to explore rose petals as an alternative worthy of sharing. When the best method to put together this romantic wrap was kindly shared with me, it turned out to be much easier than I expected.

I also sought out a more global perspective from contacts in Egypt, Mexico, Italy, and the UK, and each of their stories was a window into how our different traditions are rooted in the same spirit. Then I reached out to folks like Wiz Khalifa, Tommy Chong, Dawn Richard, Wayne Coyne, and Laganja Estranja to interview them for the book. It came as no surprise that their personal rolling stories revealed how much there is to be uncovered when we take a little extra time to look beneath the surface. Each of these conversations collectively brought me back to my joint-infused journey in China at the dawn of the millennium and reminded me again of how connection, exploration, and lightheartedness are the most essential ingredients in whatever or wherever you roll. So, if you haven't already, twist one up, take a moment to reflect, and get ready for this trip!

What Does My Rolling Style Say About Me?

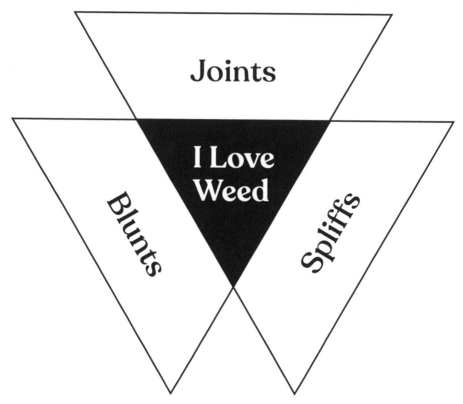

Getting Started

Put Some Prep in Your Step

Before you roll, make sure you are properly set up. You will need a good, stable surface, a rolling tray, and a grinder or a pair of scissors. If you're rolling blunts and don't want to crack them by hand, make sure to have a knife or something else sharp to cut them open. In addition, it's always good to have a tamping tool of some kind. A pencil or pen works and even a chopstick can be helpful. Now, with your army of tools and accessories perfectly parlayed, good luck finding your rolling papers.

Tray Cool, My Dude

You'll need a tray to do your magic. Take your pick from the following:

Type	Pros	Cons	Budget option
Wood or glass	Natural materials; sturdy build; Mother Earth will thank you	Heavy AF	Dinner plate/ sushi tray
Melanine/ plastic	Easy to wash; hard to break; can be used as a small sled when it snows	Over time, plastic could flake off in your weed	McDonald's™ tray/frisbee
Tin	Lightweight; easy on the wallet; can be used as a meditation gong	Prone to denting if used as a weapon	Baking sheet/ cookie tin

Cannabis Alchemy

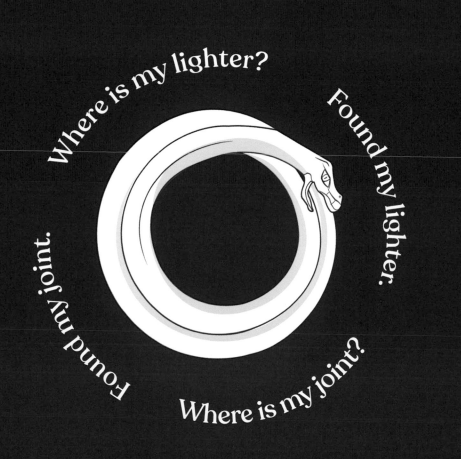

Where is my lighter?

Found my lighter.

Where is my joint?

Found my joint.

DIY Tools to Stay on the Grind

Make sure your weed is ground up before you roll up. If you're feeling too broke to buy a proper grinder, consider these options:

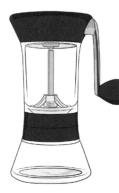

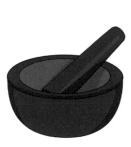

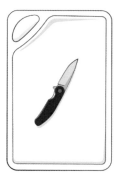

Coffee grinder

Make sure you clean out the coffee grounds before you attempt this. Fun fact: Coffee smokers are known as "bean heads."

Mortar and pestle

Put on a Gandalf hat and grind it up like a wizard from Middle Earth.

Cutting board and knife

Finally you'll get to put that culinary school degree to work!

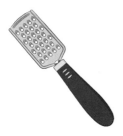

Cheese grater*

*Finger Damage Warning: Only attempt this BEFORE you've smoked weed.

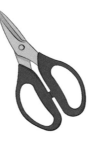

Scissors

Seriously, when was the last time you actually cut a piece of paper?

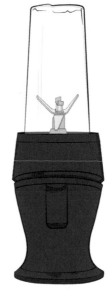

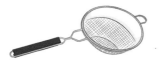

Strainer

No one will ever guess where you get that extra pesto pasta punch.

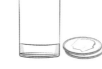

Pill bottle and coin

Shake it up and break it up while you think about how much cheaper weed is than your nasty psychiatry addiction.

Blender

You're gonna give a whole new meaning to *green juice*.

The Art of the Joint

With all kinds of options for size, materials, functionality, and beyond, joint rolling is smokin' for a reason. The first thing you need to do is pick your rolling paper. Hemp, flax, rice, and tree pulp are just a few of the plant materials you can choose from. Want an even more natural rolling experience? You can find papers that use organic fibers, natural sugar-based gum, and other wholesome materials.There's other fancy features you could consider, such as wire-in paper to make it easier to smoke down to the end or to pass to your amigos but, honestly, nothing hits quite like a classic joint.

What's the Best Way to Light a Joint?

Bic™ lighter	Classic, dependable, utilitarian.
Clipper™ lighter	Weed ninjas use the Clipper flint to pack their joints. So should you.
Hemp wick	Yes, inhaling butane kills brain cells, but so does weed, right?
Matches	Free is always the right price.
Zippo®	Rockabilly died decades ago, but apparently nostalgia never will.

Rolling Paper Sizes

Like insurance policy fine print or the electoral college, paper sizing can be extremely confusing. To make matters worse, different brands actually have slight variations in their actual measurements. The guide and chart below will (hopefully) shed some light on the matter and help you find your way.

Single wide

The single wide is narrower and typically shorter than all of the other papers on this list. This size is good for rolling a cigarette or a pinner. Generally avoid these papers if you want to roll a standard joint.

1¼

In an ideal world (preferably ruled by joint rollers), these papers would just be called "1." They are the classic, standard size of paper that fit in your hand easily and can help you roll a solid standard joint.

Double wide

The double wide paper is double the width of a 1¼ and equal in length—it's for someone who needs to roll something super fat.

1½

The 1½ is just a little bit wider and the same length as a 1¼ . Think of all the possibilities this extra real estate could offer!

84 mm

The 84 mm is like the 1¼ but just a few more millimeters in length. Measuring things in millimeters is pretty swaggy too.

King size

The king size delivers on its name. It's the same width as a 1¼ but provides more length. It's almost like a blunt wrap made of paper.

King slims

As the name suggests, if you wanna go long and narrow, this is for you. Why, might you ask? Who knows! There must be someone out there who loves these . . . salute!

Actual size:

Double wide

1 1/2

King size

King slim

84 mm

1 ¼

Single

The Birth of the Rolling Paper Is the Birth of the Joint

"You have to study the past, and learn from it, otherwise you're doomed to repeat other people's mistakes," says Josh Kesselman, CEO of RAW rolling papers. Josh has built a very public personality around sharing information about history, rolling, and other smoking-related intel. He even produces his RAW-brand papers in a traditional manner in the birthplace of rolling paper: Alcoy, Spain.

Before he digs too deep, he wants to make one thing very clear: "I think Columbus is a fucking piece of shit and I don't want to come across in any way as someone who is pro-Columbus," he says. "I think that guy is a true maniac." The reason we have no choice but to discuss Columbus, of course, is that to unpack the origins of rolling papers, we have to start with smoking's voyage to Europe, and that voyage started with Columbus.

"Native people had been smoking for perhaps thousands of years before Columbus came to the new world," says Josh. "He landed and was given cigars as a gift. He saw people smoking cigars, and he brought cigars with him back to Spain." And once the flow of tobacco began, it never ceased. Its popularity started with the upper classes who could afford it as a luxury. Josh explains, "The aristocrats would throw these juiced-up resinated remnants of tobacco and the peasants would scoop up the leftover cigars from the ground, open them up, and reroll them in newspaper. That was all anybody had back then."

In order to enjoy these scraps, peasants were unknowingly inhaling some nasty stuff, as many ingredients in the newspaper ink of that era contained harmful heavy metals. At the time, Seville was the tobacco headquarters of Spain, as decreed by the king, but as the tobacco habit spread, that evolved as well. According to Josh, when smoking out of newspapers made its way to Alcoy, Spain, "the people in Alcoy took one look at what's in that paper and they refused to do it. They turned around and made the world's first rolling paper, which was a bright white bleached paper that was designed for purity. It would have been made out of hemp like most paper was back then."

In Alcoy, their innovative attitude toward the possibilities for rolling paper stemmed from years of tradition. Alcoy had already been one of the world's capitals for paper making. Moorish conquest (and the Moors' penchant for paper producing) led them to Alcoy for its abundant supply of running water that was needed to power the early paper-making process. In addition, the climate was comparatively dry, so once the paper was produced, it could quickly air-dry and then be sold.

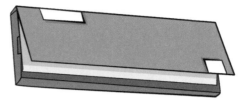

The proliferation of paper around Alcoy and the rest of Spain caused immense competition and copycat behavior among producers. So much so that when Spain opened its first trademark offices the majority of the first filings were all to protect rolling paper trademarks. In addition to this legal innovation, Josh adds, "People were copying each other to such a large extent that each maker wanted to put their mark on it, which began the habit of watermarking"—a tradition that still exists to this day on quality papers.

Alcoy was home to other rolling paper innovations, too, namely the rolling paper pack. In the early days of rolling paper, the paper itself came in giant sheets that were folded up numerous times until they were a manageable size. Smokers of the day would have to unfold the paper and tear off an individual portion and then roll their smoke. This was an inconvenience and its days were numbered. "A Dominican monk in the Alcoy region saw this and wanted to help his parishioners," says Josh. With holy intentions, "he cut the sheets and then put them into a little piece of paper. That was the first rolling paper pack."

With the evolution of rolling papers well underway, there is a logical next question to ask: With all this rolling paper innovation around, does that mean Alcoy was also the first place where somebody rolled a joint? According to Josh, the answer is an emphatic yes. "We tend to always want to give an invention to a single person, but in reality, there's probably a hundred of them," Josh responds. "My guess would be that a factory worker in Alcoy [rolled the first joint]. They were making the first rolling paper and there was so much hemp growing in Spain at the time that they were smoking the shit out of it, no question."

The birthplace of rolling papers, and (very likely) the first place someone smoked a joint, is a big legacy. It's no wonder Josh has decided to base the manufacturing of his RAW-brand papers in Alcoy with the people who have made papers for centuries. "In Alcoy, you're smacked in the face with history; it's a reminder that you're not gonna be here that long, and a lot of people did this before you," Josh reflects. With that in mind, ideas and legacy come into focus. When asked about his own perspective on creating the RAW product, Josh says, "You're not gonna make great papers with slave labor. It's got to connect people to their humanity, through love and community and art. I put that back in with passion."

"In Alcoy, you're smacked in the face with history; it's a reminder that you're not gonna be here that long, and a lot of people did this before you.... You're not gonna make great papers with slave labor. It's got to connect people to their humanity, through love and community and art. I put that back in with passion."

The Classic Joint

Everybody starts somewhere. Mozart didn't always play the piano. The Williams sisters didn't always hit blistering serves. And even the most experienced joint roller had to practice in order to master the craft. Being frustrated with yourself will not help you achieve your goal. But keeping with it, using the right tools, and believing in yourself will help guide you on your path. Visualize it now: holding a perfectly rolled joint in your hands to enjoy with yourself and others. Never forget: The magic is in your mind.

Stash Box

1 (1¼-size) rolling paper

Instructions

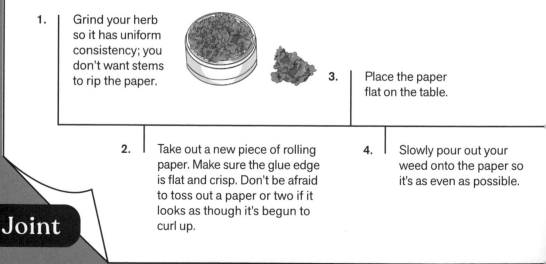

1. Grind your herb so it has uniform consistency; you don't want stems to rip the paper.

2. Take out a new piece of rolling paper. Make sure the glue edge is flat and crisp. Don't be afraid to toss out a paper or two if it looks as though it's begun to curl up.

3. Place the paper flat on the table.

4. Slowly pour out your weed onto the paper so it's as even as possible.

Joint

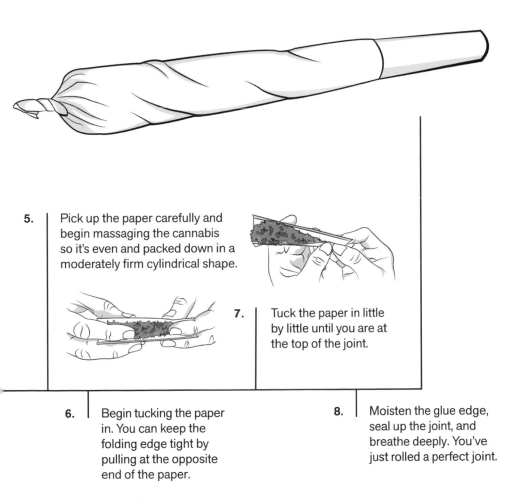

5. Pick up the paper carefully and begin massaging the cannabis so it's even and packed down in a moderately firm cylindrical shape.

7. Tuck the paper in little by little until you are at the top of the joint.

6. Begin tucking the paper in. You can keep the folding edge tight by pulling at the opposite end of the paper.

8. Moisten the glue edge, seal up the joint, and breathe deeply. You've just rolled a perfect joint.

Tommy Chong

Cheech and Chong's *Big Bambu* Album Gave Everyone a Reason to Roll

Me and Cheech were on the road because we got so popular so quickly that we were gone three months without coming home. And so Lou Adler, our producer and owner of the record company, contacted this graphic artist named Craig Braun; he was the one to come up with the big tongue logo for the Rolling Stones. Craig came up with the idea for the cover of our next album, *Big Bambu* [based on a pack of rolling papers with an actual oversize paper inside]. It was groundbreaking. We definitely sold more albums because of the cover. The paper was never meant to be smoked, but oh man, they rolled it, everybody did.

Cheech and I would sign the album all the time. And if they had the paper inside then they got what we call the three signatures—the front, the paper on the inside, and the back. And so we would always look for the paper when they'd hand us the album. And I wish we started counting them, but so many papers had a little corner torn off just the right paper size. And I don't know how many times fans have said, "Yeah, we rolled a whole pound of weed in that joint."

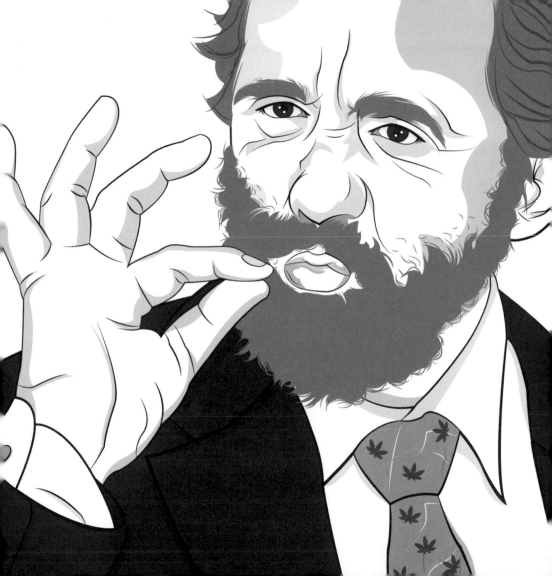

The paper company loved us too. It's a testament to who we are and to the weed itself. As soon as we did that *Bambu* album, then there was a lot of movement for the substance at the time.

When Cheech and I were together, Cheech rolled the joints. He's very artistic, and very talented. He was good and he's kind of anal too. See, with me, I don't care what it looks like, you know. I was a joint roller because that was the only way you could carry it back in the day, you know, especially the little bit of weed that we had. We used to roll those little pinners, man.

I was at a party at Lou Adler's house one time and my buddy gave me a joint full of big, old, stinky-ass Mexican skunk weed. It just was horrible. So I asked Lou where I can smoke it. He says, "Oh, go in my bedroom." So I go into Lou's bedroom and I light up the joint. I take a puff and I look over and there's John Lennon beside the bed sitting on the floor. So I say, "Hey, John, how are you doing?" I walked over and offered him a toke and he says, "Oh, no, thanks, buddy, you know, I got this immigration problem. I can't be smoking now." Then Rod Stewart walks in and goes straight for the mirror. He's fluffing out his hair, trying to make it messy. And so I offered him the smelly joint and he kind of gave it the look and said, "Nah . . . my throat." I'm quite sure they turned it down because it smelled so bad. So then I just put it out and slid it in my pocket.

As told to Noah Rubin.

Things You Can Learn From a Joint

Take your time.

Pressing harder doesn't make things better.

You can spill a little and it will be ok.

It's important to be in touch with nature.

Wetter kisses aren't always better kisses.

Sometimes you need a filter (or two).

Roll Report:

MEXICO

There's a lot more to roll up than burritos.

Fun Fact

Weed weddings started in Mexico. First noted as far back as the 1800s, leaders of the Indigenous Otomi community in Querétaro were known to get extremely blazed in order to decide if their children should get married or not. Now that's some high-level parenting!

Dank Tourist Tip

Hit up a beach in Oaxaca, like Puerto Escondido. Oaxacans grow the best weed in Mexico, which also might have something to do with their famous street food called tlayuda. It's basically a Mexican pizza. Can you argue with that?

Key Vocab

Bacha	The butt or roach of a joint
Pegarlo	Literally "to paste": putting together a joint
Gallo	Literally "a rooster": a joint
Sábana	Literally "a bed sheet": rolling paper

A Cultured Blunt

Tobacco is one of the most important plants in human history (a close tie with cannabis, obviously). Since the meeting of the old world and the new, in the middle of the last millennium (driven by exploitive European interests), tobacco has fueled global trends and trade like no other crop before or since. Its roots are in the sacred practices of Indigenous peoples of the Americas who understood, respected, and harnessed its transcendent powers. Global trade, however, transformed the plant from a sacred ally into a commodity farmed on a mass scale.

Prepare Your Blunt Like a Pro

There's nothing quite as satisfying as rolling up a blunt. Achieving a consistent roll, however, is another story. The wide variety of brands offering cigars and wraps to roll in makes each rolling technique unique. There are several categories of blunt-rolling options that are important to understand in order to roll with them proficiently. These are the main categories: blunts you can simply crack, fill, and roll; blunts with a natural leaf wrapper that needs to be carefully removed, prepped, and then smoked; and whole natural tobacco leaf that can be cut and rolled. Confused yet? There are a lot of nuances when it comes to different brands and styles of blunts, so read on and try to "wrap" your head around it.

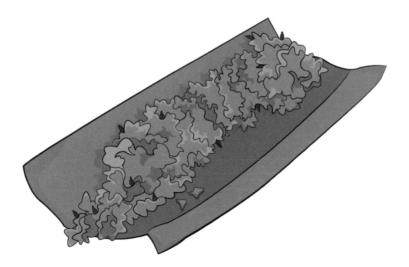

Crack and Wrap

Cigars and Cigarillos

Corner store cigars and cigarillos were first embraced by smokers in the '70s as a simple way to elevate the cannabis-smoking experience. Not only can you roll up more weed than a rolling paper, you also get the flavor and complexity of tobacco while you smoke (plus, it doesn't hurt that the strong smell of cigars can help mask the funk of your bud). The general principle here is to crack it open, empty it out, and fill it up with your favorite herb and enjoy your smoke. Look for: White Owl, Swisher Sweets, Phillies, El Producto.

Instructions

1. Put both of your thumbs on the tip of the blunt.

2. Squeeze while pulling apart gently until the wrapper begins to crack.

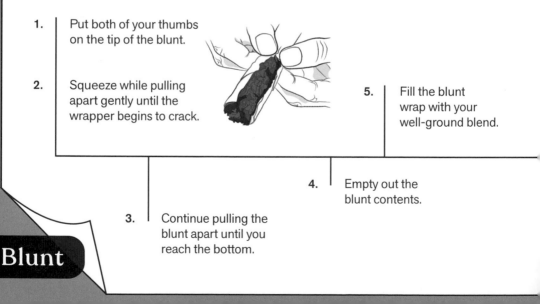

5. Fill the blunt wrap with your well-ground blend.

4. Empty out the blunt contents.

3. Continue pulling the blunt apart until you reach the bottom.

Blunt

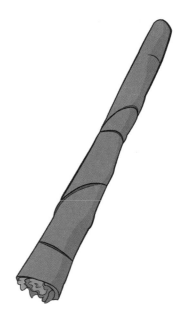

6. | Gradually compress the cannabis in the wrapper.

8. | Moisten the edge and reseal, let it dry, and then you are ready to go.

7. | Gently tuck and roll from one end to the other.

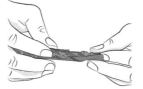

Unwrap and Roll

Leaf-Wrapped Cigars

Leaf-wrapped cigars offer an upleveled smoking experience. With a real leaf (sometimes encasing a traditional wrap), these cigars offer a lot of raw material to play with. When it comes to constructing a blunt out of a leaf-wrapped cigar, the secret is to be extra careful as you unwrap the leaf. Make sure to use a little moisture—spit, water, or even warm breath to help loosen the wrap and make it easier to unroll. Once you have unrolled the leaf, gently fill it, then roll up and enjoy! Look for: Dutch Masters, Backwoods.

Instructions

1. | Moisten the cigar with your tongue, water, or warm breath.

3. | Gently peel the leaf wrapper off the cigar.

4. | Empty out the blunt contents.

2. | Find where the seam of the tobacco wrap begins.

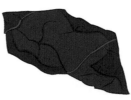

Blunt

Brand-Specific Tips

Dutch Masters: The Dutch is complicated because it has a tobacco leaf exterior plus an interior wrap. You need to carefully find the seam of the leaf, moisten it, then unwrap. Next, take the interior wrap, crack and empty it, then refill it and seal it. Finally, take the exterior leaf that you removed and reroll it around the reconstructed interior wrap.

Backwoods: Much like removing the exterior of the Dutch Masters, prepping a Backwoods for smoking takes some care and concentration. Moisten the blunt a little bit and find the end seam of the tobacco leaf. Carefully peel and unroll it, and your tobacco leaf will be ready for a roll and smoke.

5. Cut or tear the leaf into your desired size and shape.

7. Gently tuck and roll from one end to the other.

8. Moisten the edge and reseal, let it dry, toast it with a lighter to speed up drying.

6. Fill the leaf with your well-ground blend and compress.

Leafy and Beefy

Natural Tobacco Leaf

Tobacco leaf offers a very direct way to get you to your blunt enjoyment moment. Unlike other blunt-rolling options, not having to dissect a factory-rolled cigar greatly simplifies the process. That said, be careful when you tear apart the leaf and be sure to stretch it carefully or even flash-boil it to get the perfect roll. Look for: Grabba Leaf, Fronto Leafs, Funnels.

Instructions

1. Find an area of the natural leaf that does not have too many veins.

3. Some people recommend flash-boiling the leaf to clean it from mold and dirt.

2. Gently tear the leaf into a shape and size you want to roll.

4. Once the leaf is prepped, fill the blunt wrap with your well-ground blend.

Blunt

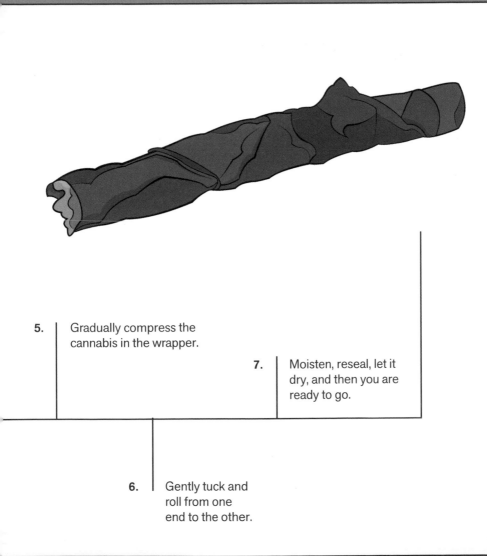

5. Gradually compress the cannabis in the wrapper.

7. Moisten, reseal, let it dry, and then you are ready to go.

6. Gently tuck and roll from one end to the other.

The Evolution of the New York City Blunt

"You know the Pope, right?" I pause for a moment. "Like, Pope Francis?" I think to myself. Who OG NYC smoker, graffiti guerilla warrior, and delivery service don Mike Saes is referring to, of course, is the infamous "Pope of Pot," Michael Cesar. "The Pope was the first big delivery service," Saes continues. "It was the early '80s, he had a phone number that was 1-800-WANT-POT, and they used to run ads on public-access TV." Now I am on page.

Of course, Saes's reminiscing about the exploits of "The Pope" is far from where NYC's weed-smoking evolution began. Uptown jazz clubs as far back as the 1920s and '30s were known haunts for weed-smoking musicians and patrons alike. Both Louis Armstrong and his weed-supplying Hebrew homie Mezz Mezzrow (born Milton Mesirow) were hitting the "gage," as they called it, years before

prohibition curbed their happy habit. Look no further than Armstrong's instrumental number "Muggles" for a prototypical stoner anthem.

Fast-forward to post-hippie New York of the 1970s, and weed culture was continuing to bubble up in the creative set. Artists, skaters, and other pioneers of early NYC street culture came together in the parks to get out of their families' cramped apartments and engage in the buzz of city life. "Anybody that hung out in the Central Park bandshell back in those days knows about dollar joints," Saes offers. He's referring, of course, to the most common format for buying weed on the street in that era: a pre-rolled joint that cost one dollar. Places like the Central Park bandshell and Washington Square Park were hotbeds of cultural activity where many future legends would come together for a hang and a smoke, sanctifying the intersection of cannabis and street culture.

As the '70s gave way to the '80s, the one-dollar joint was eclipsed by new innovations. "We used to go out to Myrtle on the G train to buy tré bags," Saes says. "That was three dollars of weed in a manila envelope." The new format not only provided more revenue for dealers but also put the creativity of the rolling process in the hands of New York City cannabis consumers. Saes reflects, "I smoked my first blunt in '82, but I'm sure I wasn't the first person to smoke one." Alongside rolling innovation, slang evolved as well. Because early NYC blunt smokers often gravitated toward El Producto cigars, the classic question "Do you want to smoke an L?" (or "El," as the case may be) still permeates stoner lingo.

Once the '80s were in full swing, NYC dealers continued to up their game. The birth of dime and nickel bags (ten and five dollars, respectively) gave smokers even more material to work with. Savvy smokers could cop a "chicken sack"–an overstuffed bag of weed sold at certain spots that could easily be broken down into numerous dime or nickel bags and then sold while still allowing some leftovers for personal smoking. In addition, the proliferation of delivery services meant weed on demand was becoming a reality for all.

At the same time, harder drugs began hitting the city, and smokers reacted by mixing these drugs with their blunts and joints. "That was a bad phase of weed smoking," says Saes. "Coolies" were joints laced with cocaine, and "Woolies" were blunts laced with crack. He adds, "You would smoke a blunt and you wouldn't know if there was crack in it." For broke artists and street kids too, adding angel dust to blunts offered a way for them to get higher for less money. This hard-drug era ravaged young minds and vulnerable communities but also birthed a new generation of urban artists. These artists drew from the grit of street experiences and became part of cultural movements that influenced the globe—not only with the power of their art and music but also with the possibilities of smoking a fat New York City–style blunt.

"Music always makes things trendy," says Saes. And late '80s/early '90s rap pushed the trend of blunt smoking to a whole new level. Staten Island rap group Wu-Tang Clan took the world by storm while referencing White Owls and Dutch Masters in their rhymes. And it wasn't just about rolling standard blunts, either. A quick listen to Queensbridge's own Nas on his song

"Music always makes things trendy."

"Suspect" from 1996 reveals his reference to the "Siamese blunt," a method of putting two Phillies blunt wrappers together to create a more massive smoke.

Trends in music were mirrored in street fashion. Tapping into the blunt wave, NYC graffiti artists Gerb, Futura, and Stash, with their nascent streetwear brand GFS, started producing T-shirts with the Phillies Blunt logo front and center. The shirts were immediately embraced by rappers and musicians who wore them while performing live and on TV. The shirts were also embraced by countless bootleggers who proliferated the design on street corners everywhere. The blunt-driven style trend was born and it led to an official license of the design for GFS from Phillies and the further global onslaught of blunt-rolling culture.

This peak moment for blunts also opened the door for more influences and revisions beyond traditional blunt-smoking methods. Smokers in NYC who had connections to West Indian traditions began using Fronto Leaves—a full uncut tobacco leaf that could be used to roll numerous blunts. Other people veered away from smoking with tobacco altogether as the '90s ushered in health consciousness among smokers. "One day I was like, yo, we gotta stop rolling blunts," says Saes. "We thought we would

get tongue cancer from licking the tobacco." Having avoided any major health consequences from his smoking, however, he laughs and says, "It's funny, I feel like weed counteracts everything . . . ."

Moving into the 2000s and beyond, NYC blunt-smoking trends simultaneously embraced the future, the past, and the world at large. From putting glass tips in blunts to using see-through cellophane wraps and, more recently, using CBD-infused hemp wrappers, NYC blunt smokers know no boundaries when it comes to enhancing the smoking experience. Alongside these new traditions, rolling up a Dutch Masters remains a mainstay of New York smoking culture. The Fronto tradition from decades before has recently been updated with the trend of adding Jamaican "grabba" (tobacco leaf) to joints. As in many places, the saying also definitely applies here: The more things change, the more things stay the same. And as Saes adds, it doesn't hurt that "the weed is really, really that good."

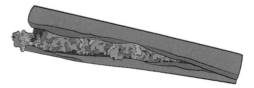

AST-ROLL-OGY

What to Roll, According to the Stars

Aries
March 21–April 19

Ruling Planet: Mars
Symbol: Ram
Recommended Roll: Pinner joint

Analysis: As the first sign of the horoscope, Aries is sometimes considered the baby. Always eager and occasionally competitive, you need to roll something that is in tune with your occasionally delicate disposition. Start small and roll a pinner joint.

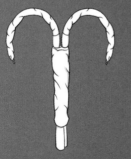

Taurus
April 20–May 20

Ruling Planet: Venus
Symbol: Bull
Recommended Roll: Cannon

Analysis: Taurus season starts on 4/20, so you definitely have to be rolling something legit. Channel your strength and dependability to roll up a fat cannon joint, 'cause you know everyone in the room is gonna be ready for a hit!

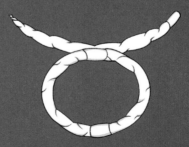

Gemini

May 21–June 20

Ruling Planet: Mercury

Symbol: Twins

Recommended Roll: Shotgun joint

Analysis: Gemini is the twin: Double the pleasure, double the fun, everyone knows two joints are better than one! Put twin rolls together in a shotgun joint to best savor your dualistic personality.

Cancer

June 21–July 22

Ruling Planet: Moon

Symbol: Crab

Recommended Roll: Spliff

Analysis: The protective cancer is sometimes hesitant to share with outsiders. Roll a classic spliff, scurry back to your comfy cave, and enjoy a bit of solitude.

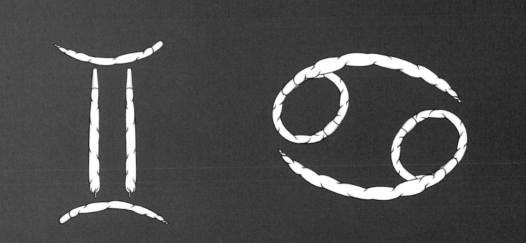

Leo

July 23–August 22

Ruling Planet: Sun

Symbol: Lion

Recommended Roll: L Paper Joint

Analysis: Leo is known for generosity, especially among friends and family, but also has a bit of a narcissistic streak. Grab two papers and roll up an L paper joint for an extra-friendly Leo-themed smoke.

Virgo

August 23– September 22

Ruling Planet: Mercury

Symbol: The Virgin (Mary)

Recommended Roll: Classic joint

Analysis: Flawless presentation and exacting detail are no stranger to Virgo. Roll a perfectly tucked classic joint and wait for the haters to claim you used a rolling machine.

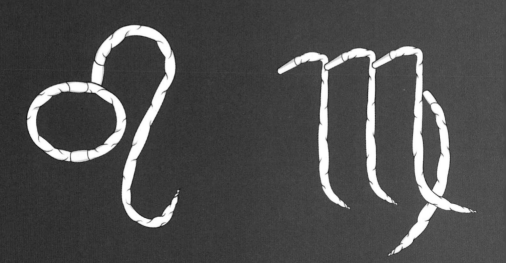

Libra
September 23–October 22

Ruling Planet: Venus

Symbol: Scales

Recommended Roll: Crack and wrap blunt

Analysis: Libras are known for always considering every side of a situation, but Libra is also the only sign of the zodiac symbolized by a natural weed accessory—the scale! Take a moment to kick back, weigh out some of your best weed, and roll up a crack and wrap–style blunt.

Scorpio
October 23–November 21

Ruling Planet(s): Mars/Pluto

Symbol: Scorpion

Recommended Roll: Scorpion joint

Analysis: A passionate and sometimes stubborn Scorpio should never hesitate to celebrate themselves. Assemble a scorpion joint and ponder what it's like to smoke yourself . . .

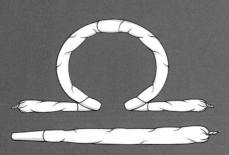

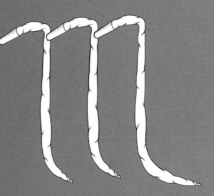

Sagittarius

November 22–December 21

Ruling Planet: Jupiter

Symbol: Centaur

Recommended Roll: Hash and cannabis–blended spliff

Analysis: Sagittarians are fearless explorers of the world. Show off your international flair with an Italian-style "primavera" spliff (page 131).

Capricorn

December 22–January 19

Ruling Planet: Saturn

Symbol: Horned sea-goat

Recommended Roll: Natural leaf blunt

Analysis: Determination and discipline come naturally for Capricorn, which definitely helps when you are crafting the perfect roll. Carefully prepare a natural tobacco leaf and roll up a full-flavored blunt!

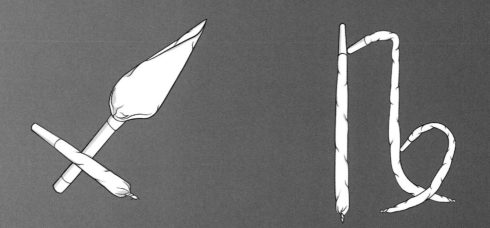

Aquarius

January 20–February 18

Ruling Planet(s): Saturn/Uranus

Symbol: Water bearer

Recommended Roll: Twax rolled, kief-dipped joint

Analysis: Aquarians love to share their deep originality with the world. Don't fear the flashiness: Roll up a kief-covered, twax-twirled joint and let the world take note!

Pisces

February 19–March 20

Ruling Planet(s): Jupiter/Neptune

Symbol: Two fish

Recommended Roll: Pipe joint

Analysis: Pisces embodies the spirit of water and the ocean with overflowing empathy and artistic vibes. Put together a pipe joint, take a few puffs, and make Popeye proud.

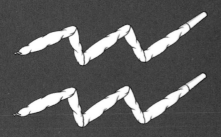

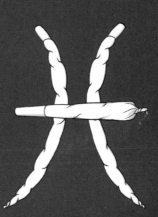

When Music Legends Are Cool About Smoking a Joint

Dr. Dre ft. Snoop Dogg - "Still D.R.E."

Just because Dre's verse was reportedly written by Jay-Z doesn't mean it isn't one of his most smoking tracks of all time.

Ozzy Osbourne on Black Sabbath's - "Sweet Leaf"

Ozzy loved the sweet leaf long before he loved reality TV.

Miley Cyrus - "Dooo It!"

Miley's collaboration with the Flaming Lips is a smoker's gem.

OutKast - "Crumblin' Erb"

Increase the peace by rolling one up, duh.

When the Same Legends Aren't Cool About Smoking a Joint

Dr. Dre. on NWA's - "Express Yourself"

Dre dissing weed is like soda dissing bubbles.

Ozzy Osbourne - "Straight to Hell"

Ozzy teams up with Guns N' Roses members for an ANTI-drug song, proving again that 2020 was one of the weirdest years ever.

Miley Cyrus - "Slide Away"

Letting go is hard to do, especially if it's a really good joint.

OutKast - "Git Up, Git Out"

Smoke joints to be chill, but not enough to make you lazy AF.

Roll Report:

EGYPT

Camel humps are Mother Nature's stash spot.

Fun Fact

Hash and cannabis smoking is a multigenerational pastime in Egypt, even though most Egyptians don't discuss it openly. Alcohol is directly prohibited in Islam, but cannabis is not specifically forbidden and enjoys a gray-area status as a result. Older Egyptians can be found in social clubs adding hash to their gozah (hookah) for a little extra kick, while younger Egyptians stick mostly to rolling joints and spliffs.

Dank Tourist Tip

There's no way you're going to Egypt and not seeing a pyramid, but if the crowds at Giza sound like a buzzkill, put in an extra few minutes of travel time to visit the pyramids at Saqqâra. Saqqâra and its famous Pyramid of Djoser offer a mellow way to enjoy mystical and mysterious structures that were built (by aliens?) almost five thousand years ago. Don't forget to ponder ancient Egyptians' cannabis use while you roll one up.

Key Vocab

Maktab or marral	Literally "desk" or "roller": a piece of paper used to mix tobacco and hash
Cartela	Literally "a little card": a paper filter tip
Fabric	A cheaper, modern type of hash that is lighter to smoke
Job	A joint
Bafra	Rolling paper

Superior Spliffs

For most of the world outside of the United States, the most common way to roll up and smoke cannabis is alongside tobacco. But that doesn't mean there aren't places in the States that also enjoy mixing the two. From a hash spliff in a Dutch coffee shop to the infamous sheets and funnels in the DMV (a.k.a. DC, Maryland, and Virginia), harnessing the power of these plants together sometimes means that 1 + 1 can equal 3. It also underlines the important historical relationship between the development of cannabis rolling styles alongside tobacco-related technologies and techniques.

Get to Know a Spliff

Type	Pros	Cons
Hash and tobacco	A little cube of hash is easy to stash.	High school Amsterdam vacay flashbacks. So spinyyyyyy.
Cannabis and tobacco	The fun never ends when you master the blend.	Canna connoisseurs will accuse you of ruining their greens.
Cannabis, hash, and tobacco	It's perfecta when you roll with the trifecta.	Too much hash and you're on your ass.
Cannabis and grabba	Feel like a chief when you roll with the leaf.	Too many puffs feels like smoking the tailpipe of a Mack Truck.

Where Are My Rolling Papers?

In My Car
12.5%

In My
Other Jacket
12.5%

In My
Stash Box
12.5%

Right in
Front of Me on
the Table
37.5%

Up in Smoke
25%

Country Songs
About Smoking Weed. . .

. . . Not by Willie Nelson	. . . By Willie Nelson	. . . With Willie Nelson
"High Time" Kacey Musgraves	"It's All Going to Pot" with Merle Haggard	"Weed with Willie" Toby Keith
"Weed Instead of Roses" Ashley Monroe	"Roll Me Up and Smoke Me When I Die"	"Weed, Whiskey and Willie" Brothers Osborne
"Get High" Brandy Clark	"My Medicine" with Snoop Dogg	"Willie Nelson's Wall" Eleven Hundred Springs
"Smoke a Little Smoke" Eric Church		
"Might as Well Get Stoned" Chris Stapleton		
"Sun Daze" Florida Georgia Line		

Natural Leaves

If tobacco isn't your speed and rolling papers feel like a bore, then a natural leaf–rolling option might be for you. There's lots of good reasons to experiment: Different smoking flavors, cleaner mouthfeel, and better overall cannabis taste are just a few. It's important to note that not all of these will offer a healthier alternative, so consider that in your selection process.

Cannagar

That's right, take some magical cannabis leaves, press up some cannabis around a stick like a skunky, green kebob, roll it up, and you are ready to go! Double the pleasure, double the fun!

Rose petals

Roses aren't just for Valentine's Day, but they still can be if your special someone loves smoking weed as much as you. Take some rose petals and press them together for a sublime, smooth, and potentially romantic puff.

Tendu leaf (beedi)

In India the beedi is a very popular way to smoke tobacco, but the same leaf can make a great wrapper for cannabis as well. Sweet, pungent, and easy to find in tobacco stores, this leaf should definitely be in your arsenal.

Banana leaf

Who isn't bananas for bananas? Especially banana leaves full of weed, ya know?

Corn husk

Corn, corn, everywhere there's corn. Corn is everywhere, and now you know that you can actually use the husk to roll up your weed. What could be better? Bonus idea: Corn husk can be cut and folded to make a very competent filter tip.

Cordia leaf

Cordia is an amazingly regenerative plant that can provide an eco-conscious way to smoke weed with a full, smooth flavor. Many wraps marketed as "palm leaves" are actually cordia leaves, FYI.

Lomboy

Lumpia are traditional Fillipino fried spring rolls. Fillipino lomboy leaf, on the other hand, provides a whole different kind of roll. Traditionally found in open-air markets, lomboy is often smoked with tobacco but can easily be adapted for your favorite herbal concoction.

Rose Petals

What is more poetic and inspiring than a rose? Especially when it is full of some top-notch herb? This subtle twist on a classic roll-up is guaranteed to turn heads. How many people have ever seen a rose joint? Frankly, not many. And even the most hesitant smoker will want to check out what you've cooked up. It also makes a great Valentine's Day gift. And who doesn't love that?

Stash Box

6 to 10 rose petals

Instructions

1. Take two flattened, semi–dry rose petals. Lick the edge of one and stick it to the other so they form a heart shape.

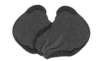

3. Let dry for about 3 minutes.

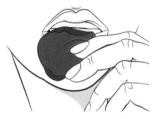

2. Repeat step 1 until all of your petals are stuck together in pairs of two.

4. Lick the tip (pointed side of the "heart") of one of your petal pairs and stick it to the top of another one of your petal pairs (rounded side of the "heart") and repeat until all the petals are stuck together.

Joint

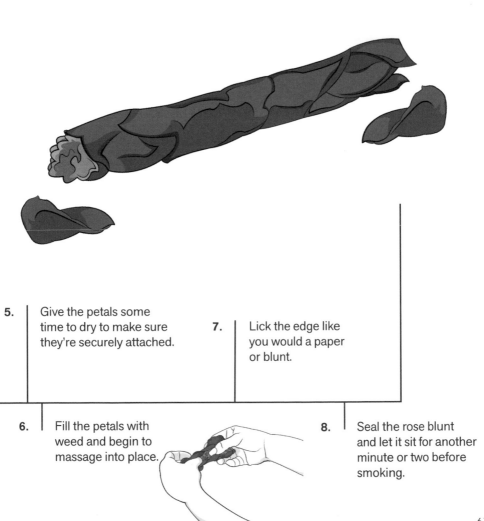

5. Give the petals some time to dry to make sure they're securely attached.

7. Lick the edge like you would a paper or blunt.

6. Fill the petals with weed and begin to massage into place.

8. Seal the rose blunt and let it sit for another minute or two before smoking.

Dawn Richard

From NOLA to New York on a Cloud of Cannabis

I came from a very strict Southern home; my parents were devout Catholics. I didn't know anything about cannabis until I left New Orleans and was actually in the music industry and moved to New York when I was on *Making the Band*, especially because I was signed to a hip-hop label. In the studio with Bad Boy everybody smoked. When you walked out of Studio A, it was clouds of smoke coming out of the studio, you got a contact high just from being in the space. And before you know it, you're like, OK, this is a vibe. Art and cannabis go hand in hand and I got open to a whole new world just by being a part of it.

When you go into the studio, there's at least one professional roller that only is there to roll everybody's blunt. They were always rolling with big Backwoods. It was wild to watch; there was an art to it that I just always appreciated because every time I would try to roll, I failed miserably. It's also crazy because, like I said, coming from the South where people snuck around to do that, I promise you, I never was exposed to any of that.

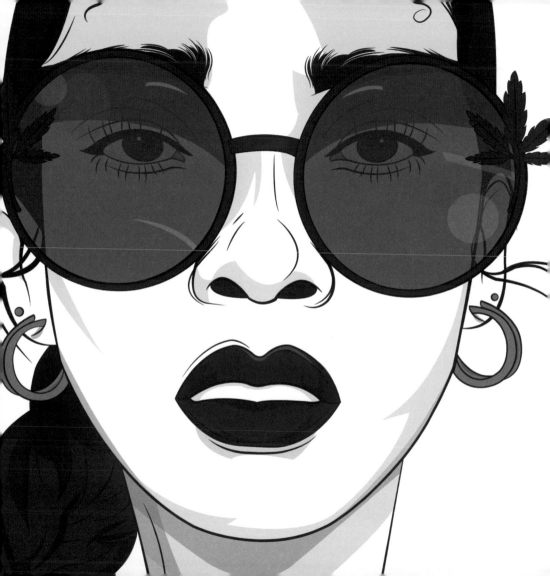

The best weed session of my entire life, no question, was Grace Jones. We were doing "Yeah Yeah You Would" for the Dirty Money project. It was me, Kalenna, and Grace and we were vocal-producing Grace for the record. She had a bottle of red wine and a blunt and that's how we started the session. And when I tell you she was amazing, she was high off her ass and she sounded like a beautiful black ocean.

Puff didn't even come until later, so we really had an intimate time. We talked about men; we talked about sex. It was just so much shit talking and so much chocolate in the studio. We went through two bottles of wine and two bags of weed. She's Jamaican, so there was a level of like, she's an island girl at heart . . . it was just a cool-ass vibe. It was one of those out-of-body experiences for me. I wasn't prepared for it to be a real smoke session or to be with a legend. That's forever going to be the best cannabis experience I've ever been a part of.

Later, when I realized cannabis could also be a holistic journey, that's when I really fell in love with it. I grew up with fibroid tumors. You get severe cramps and severe pain when you have your journey every month. And I tried everything, it was really bad. I was reading up that cannabis could save you. People have used it for cancer.

They've used it through pain issues. And I thought, well, let me try the flower and see what works for me. And it was one of the best months of my life because I was not in pain for the first time ever. I realized that there was another way instead of me taking all these different medications. As time has progressed, it's been really cool to see what cannabis was for me in the very beginning and how it has evolved.

As told to Noah Rubin.

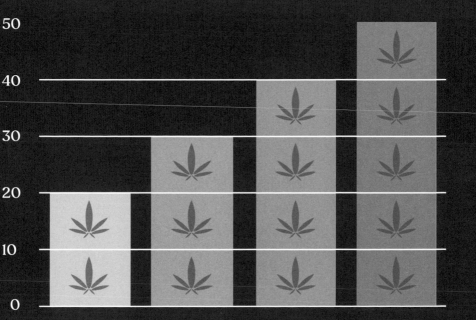

Age				
50				
40				
30				
20				
10				
0	What people around me are listening to	What people younger than me are listening to	Nature sounds on YouTube	Actual nature

Wraps, Cellulose, and Other Plant Blends

Sometimes you don't wanna roll with paper or tobacco or even other natural leaves and fibers. The options listed on the next page are often made of reconstituted natural materials and can offer consistent smokability as well as interesting flavors and looks.

Gold leaf

Do you love to order bottle service at the club, with sparklers blaring and a procession of waiters delivering your goods? If so, smoking 24-karat-gold blunt wraps might be for you!

Cellulose

If you can't be clearheaded, at least be clear-blunted. Cellulose wraps are a completely transparent and smokable wrap that looks almost like Saran wrap. Not recommended for your grandma's leftovers, however.

Mint

It's always good to keep things minty fresh, and minty wraps are proof. Whether you want a menthol-like smoking experience (Newport lovers, I'm looking at you) or just like the idea of smoking out of a mint leaf–blended wrap, these can give you a very refreshing roll.

Hemp

It all comes back to the source, and hemp wraps are one of the most convenient and reliable ways to roll up and smoke your cannabis. In addition, hemp has naturally occurring CBD that some people believe can help counteract certain negative effects of smoking.

Tips and Filters

Here's a tip: From glass to paper to natural fibers to cigarette-style filters, adding a tip to your roll can add not only convenience of roll but also smoothness of smoke.

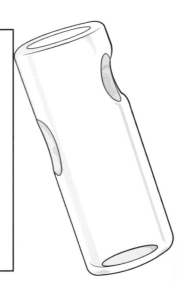

Glass

Glass can make smoking taste smoother and can also add some visual appeal to your roll if you choose colored or chameleon glass. But glass can be a little bit slippery to roll with, so beware!

Paper tip/cone

Paper tips will help you hold on to your blunt or joint right down to the last ember without risk of burning your fingers. In addition, paper tips can help guide you in making a cone-shaped roll, if that's what you want to do. If you don't want to buy cardboard tips at the store, lots of household paper, especially business cards, can be a great DIY option for getting your roll on.

Cigarette-style filters

This style of filter can smooth out even the harshest smoke. If you are rolling something with tobacco mixed in, it can reduce the amount of tar that you inhale and make you less prone to coughing. The other side of that coin, however, is that when smoking cannabis through this type of filter, it will likely reduce the amount of THC (or CBD) your body is getting.

Roll a Proper Tip

Not all tips are created equal. Below are four great filter tip–rolling options. The secret is to roll them tightly both ways, creating tension on each side of the paper so it doesn't spring outward and lose tension when you complete your roll.

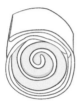

The spiral:

This is a great tip for first-timers: Just roll the paper tightly in one direction, then release. Next, unroll the tip and roll the paper tightly in the opposite direction, and release. Now you have a nice, concise spiral for your joint.

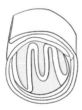

The M:

Start by making one small fold (about 1 mm) in the paper, then fold it back on itself. Fold it back on itself again (both about 1 mm) and release. If you did this right, the end of the paper should resemble an *M*. Next, roll the tip up tightly from the non-folded side. Then roll the folded *M* side tightly all the way to the end and release. Mmmmmm so good . . .

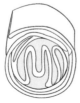

The M+M:

Start like you did with the *M* but with with six folds instead of three. Sadly, there is no milk chocolate or peanut option.

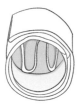

The hollow:

Follow the *M+M* instructions from the previous page, but before you begin rolling in either direction, cut out half of the folded section with a pair of scissors. First cut halfway down the last fold in your second *M,* and then cut down the middle of the folded section to meet the first cut you made. Now roll up the folded section the same as above and you will see that the tip is hollow on one end.

Tips for DIY Tips

DO	DON'T
Use medium–thick new paper	Use anything printed with a lot of ink
Neatly cut or tear the paper so it can be rolled easily	Use anything too thin
Place your tip at the end of your rolling paper to guide your roll	Use any paper you're afraid of damaging, like those Grateful Dead ticket stubs from New Year's Eve '79

A Cone and a Cannon

Once you've mastered the subtle art of rolling a tip, it's time to put that knowledge to work. Grab a paper, prep a tip, and slip it in. Stay focused as you gently shape the joint with your hands. You want to roll it straight on for a cannon or at an angle for a cone. Tuck it in, seal it up, and you're ready to go!

Stash Box

1 (1¼- or king-size) rolling paper
1 angled paper tip (for a cone) or 1 straight paper tip (for a cannon)

Instructions

1. Place a piece of rolling paper in front of you on the table.

2. Roll your preferred tip and put it on one end.

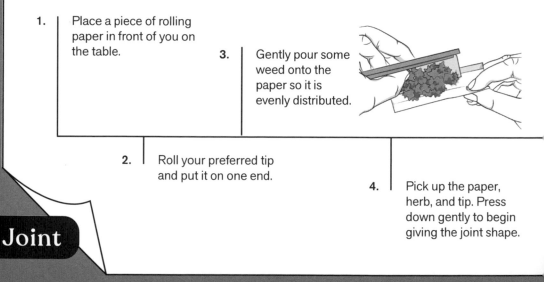

3. Gently pour some weed onto the paper so it is evenly distributed.

4. Pick up the paper, herb, and tip. Press down gently to begin giving the joint shape.

Joint

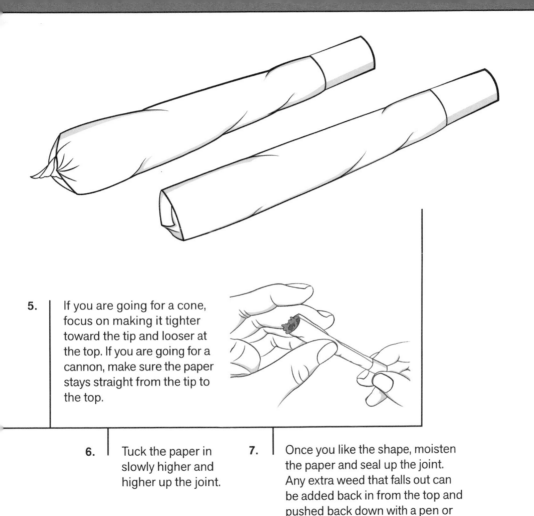

5. If you are going for a cone, focus on making it tighter toward the tip and looser at the top. If you are going for a cannon, make sure the paper stays straight from the tip to the top.

6. Tuck the paper in slowly higher and higher up the joint.

7. Once you like the shape, moisten the paper and seal up the joint. Any extra weed that falls out can be added back in from the top and pushed back down with a pen or other tool.

Trinidad Smokes the Funk

Trinidad is home to magical beaches, beautiful blue ocean, and a complex history indicative of the Caribbean's role in the birth of transatlantic commerce and the legacy of the slave trade. It's also home to one of the most interesting rolling traditions anywhere in the world. The Trinidadian "roll on" is a hybrid joint that in many ways embodies the layered cultural history of the island itself. The construction of this specialty joint involves breaking a cigarette in two, leaving about 1 inch of the tobacco in front of the filter, and then rolling a full joint around the stub of tobacco. As you smoke the joint, the cigarette portion absorbs the THC-filled resin and provides an extra-long experience for the smoker.

Marcus Ramkissoon is one of Trinidad's foremost authorities on cannabis, having helped numerous countries in the West Indies draft medical cannabis legislation. He is also an unexpected ambassador for Trinidad's roll on. Through his global travels and multitude of connections, he has made the roll on a vehicle of awareness for both his story and this island-original rolling technique. He's the ideal guide to understanding both the technicalities and the history of this funky joint.

There's more to it than simply a joint and part of a cigarette rolled together. Trinidadians describe sections of the roll on with special terminology like "the top of the world" and "the funk." Marcus explains, "The 'top of the world' is where the cannabis and the cigarette meet," adding, "that last inhalation where you get both raw cannabis and some tobacco is regarded as the best pull of the roll on."

But once a smoker has enjoyed the "top of the world," there is more to appreciate. As Marcus says, "When you smoke a pure joint and stick the cigarette in and extend it into a roll on, the resin now has more place to move and goes straight through into the cigarette. It frees up the space and you have something more to smoke than a single joint." And when asked what that resin-filled cigarette is called, Marcus quickly replies, "We just say 'funk.'"

With a basic understanding of Trinidad's roll on, one can delve deeper into the layered sociopolitical, economic, and anthropological origins of the world's funkiest smoke. One of the key elements to understand when it comes to any Caribbean smoking tradition, Jamaica included, is that cannabis came to the West Indies via indentured servants who were brought from India as a source of cheap labor for European business interests in the mid-1800s. With increasing awareness of slavery's moral depravity and its eventual prohibition, Indian laborers were in high demand, and as they arrived in the West Indies, they brought their ganja-smoking tradition with them. *Ganja* is the Hindu word for cannabis, though in the West it is most often associated with Jamaican slang. This linguistic nuance is just one by-product of Indian laborers sharing their weed-smoking habits with other local Caribbean workers in need of herbal relief.

Ganja was widely accepted by working people in the West Indies of all backgrounds, and so as different economic tides affected their lives, so did their consumption patterns. Marcus traces that correlation to the early development of the roll on. "I think that the major reason it started in Trinidad was really conservation," he says. "During the time of the Second World War, Trinidad was in a state of real depression. People had no money and the economy dropped; everything would have been hard. Rolling a joint on a cigarette would help people get enough of a smoke to get them a little higher and to stretch what they have."

Marcus's in-depth thinking around the origin of the roll on and general passion for cannabis have both been integral in opening doors for him and also bringing awareness to this smoking style worldwide. "When I went to Amsterdam for the first time, the roll was what attracted most people to talk to us," says Marcus. But it turns out it wasn't just anyone he was talking to. When riding a shuttle bus to the Amsterdam Cannabis Cup in 2008, Marcus had a chance encounter with legendary grower, breeder, smoker, and star of the infamous show *Strain Hunters*, Franco Loja.

Marcus explains that when Franco, who passed away in 2017, saw him smoke the roll on, he "laughed a little bit. Like, what!? What's that???"

The seed that Marcus planted in Franco's mind bloomed a year later when Marcus returned again to Amsterdan and visited Franco's home base, the Green House Coffeeshop. Upon walking into the shop, Franco immediately recognized Marcus and demanded that he join him for a meeting with Franco's partner in Green House and co-star on *Strain Hunters,* Arjan Roskam. "Arjan and Franco came in, sat me down in their coffee shop and said, 'Look, we want to do an episode of *Strain Hunters* in Trinidad,'" says Marcus. "It's the roll on that brought that on."

When the *Strain Hunters* crew made it down to film in Trinidad and the neighboring island of Saint Vincent (widely known for its top–tier outdoor cannabis cultivation), it was Marcus's roll on that again brought the vibes. Between exploring weed grows in the mountains and checking out local hang spots, Marcus recalls Franco's passion for the roll on. "We spent ten days in very close quarters, and as soon as he would see me walking in, he'd say, 'Eh, roll a roll on, alright?'" Marcus's specialty roll is a key element of the episode they filmed, and it

has been viewed millions of times online, spreading the gospel of this truly singular rolling style.

In the years since the release of the *Strain Hunters* Trinidad episode, Marcus has seen the roll on continue to proliferate. "Everybody I meet outside of Trinidad, even within the Caribbean, is amazed at the roll on," he says. There's something magnetic and undeniable about the roll. You might even say that the "funk" and the "top of the world" have truly conquered all. Marcus adds with a sense of pride mixed with happy surprise, "People now do this all over . . . they send me videos from all over the world."

"The 'top of the world' is where the cannabis and the cigarette meet... that last inhalation where you get both raw cannabis and some tobacco is regarded as the best pull of the roll on."

Movies Where the Kids Smoke a Joint (or Two)

FAST TIMES AT RIDGEMONT HIGH (1982)

Sean Penn's Spicoli character proves the importance of
getting pizza delivered straight to your history class.

THE BREAKFAST CLUB (1985)

Saturday school detention is beyond terrible, but not as
bad if you roll one up in the library.

DAZED AND CONFUSED (1993)

Smoking cannabis can open your mind to seeing the world in new ways . . .
or it can lead to flimsy theories about George Washington's toking habits.

SCARY MOVIE (2000) + SCARY MOVIE 2 (2001)

The only thing stronger than weed that makes you see dead people
is weed so powerful that instead of you rolling it, it rolls you!

Movies Where the Adults Smoke a Joint (or Two)

POLTERGEIST (1982)

Long before you could Netflix and chill, you would watch the tube and smoke a doob.

AMERICAN BEAUTY (1999)

The two-thousand-dollar-per-ounce government-engineered weed plotline pushes this film from insightful commentary to eye-rolling fictional exaggeration.

IT'S COMPLICATED (2009)

Who knew a single hit could get someone so lit . . . just ask Meryl Streep!

BAD TEACHER (2011)

Are we really supposed to believe that Cameron Diaz wants to get breast implants to win the affection of a character played by Justin Timberlake? What were these writers smoking???

Fight for Cannabis Justice in Less Time Than It Takes to Roll a Joint

If you know your stuff, it should take you three to five minutes to roll a joint, blunt, or spliff. In that same amount of time, you could also help change the lives of people who have been victims of the war on drugs. Just ask Weldon Angelos, founder of the Weldon Project and Mission [Green], who has set his sights on doing just that by helping free prisoners serving outlandish sentences for cannabis-related crimes. Outlandish sentencing is something Weldon knows too much about—as an emerging hip-hop producer in the early 2000s, Weldon got busted by the Salt Lake City Police for selling weed and was sentenced to fifty-five years in prison. Thanks to high-profile support from folks like senators Cory Booker, Mike Lee, and Rand Paul, as well as entertainers like Snoop, Alicia Keys, Bonnie Raitt, and Mike Epps, Weldon was granted clemency by President Obama and received a full pardon from President Trump. Now a free man, he is helping others who suffered like he did. Here are some tips from Weldon on how you too can roll with the movement and get involved.

Get Informed About the Issue

Research organizations that specialize in these issues so you can understand what's happening and what you can do about it. The Weldon Project has stories on its website that people can go through to educate themselves. You can find out why a person is in prison, what happened to them, and what it takes to get them out of jail, as well as what it takes to change a particular law or to help this person individually.

Vote

We decide how our lives are run through the people we send to DC, especially members of Congress who make the laws that we have to live with. A lot of people think that they can't do anything by voting, but your vote matters. You don't have to vote on a party line; vote on the person, their record, and what they stand for. Support the candidates that believe in ending this unjust war on cannabis.

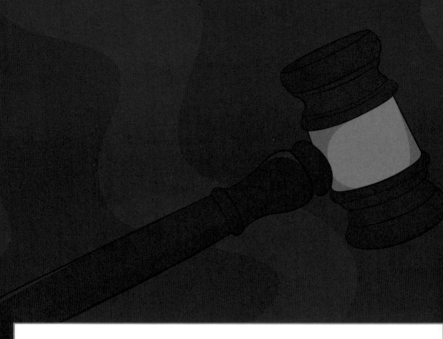

Donate and Shop Smart

Donate to the cause by supporting nonprofits that are doing important work. The more funding they have, the more resources they can bring to the table: more lawyers, more attorney work, more PR. You can also purchase products where a percentage goes to the cause.

Call Your Representatives in Congress

Call your congressperson and tell them it's time we end prohibition so people don't have to worry about being incarcerated for cannabis ever again. We need both sides to pass laws in the Senate, so it's important that Republican senators and Republican members of Congress are supportive of this kind of legislation. If we can get certain states on board, we actually have a realistic likelihood of passing this kind of reform.

Share Knowledge

You'd be surprised how many cannabis users don't know that people are still in prison for cannabis. There are people serving thirty years, forty years, sometimes life. Taking the time to share stories and educate the community about these injustices can help change public opinion.

Places You Don't Wanna Get Caught Smoking a Joint

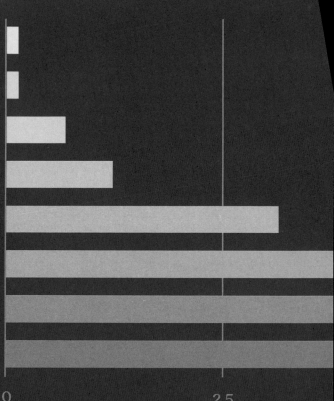

China

Russia

Saudi Arabia

Venezuela

Serbia

United Arab Emirates

Japan

Singapore

Years in Prison   0   2.5

Help Victims of the War on Drugs

There are a number of programs for people getting out, especially those with cannabis-related offenses. The majority of people that come out of prison want to be successful, but they need the tools and access to the right help so they can reintegrate successfully.

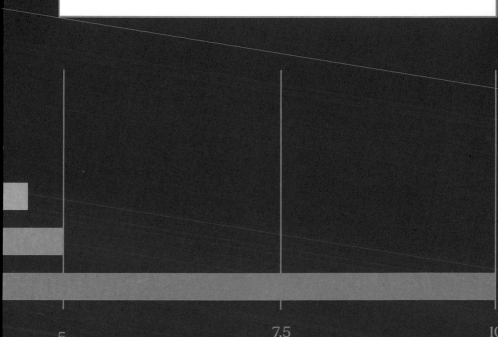

5   7.5   10

Swami: Real Joint Knowledge from the Last Hippie Standing

The sun is just peeking over the horizon in

Swami hasn't always been the face of a

the California craft cannabis movement and the roller/inventor of a signature joint style that offers an unparalleled smoking experience. Lovingly referred to as simply a "Swami joint," its impressive girth and consistent smoke are the offspring of years of refinement and evolution.

"The smoking experience is about stopping, pausing, and savoring the flavor of whatever it is you're smoking," muses Swami. He is sitting on the porch of his mountain ranch home, overlooking the cannabis garden and relaxing after the first day of this year's harvest. He's also enjoying a smoke with one of his signature joints. "It becomes almost religious as well, where you say, 'OK, I'm stopping the regular flow and now I'm into my cannabis flow.'" And when it comes to cannabis flow, Swami is an expert, blending experiences with hippie culture, Eastern spirituality, cannabis cultivation, as well as cannabis judging to bring a multifaceted perspective on enjoying cannabis that is so evolved it does in fact hint at the sacred.

"Michoacan, Acapulco Gold, and Panama Red—those are the first appellations that I knew of as a hippie," he says. Sitting back in his chair, he takes another puff and reflects on a typical day with his hippie commune companions. "We would sit down in the morning, have a cup of espresso, and roll up fifteen or twenty joints with a Rizla roller." He continues, "We would get in the Volkswagen van and we'd go out to Golden Gate Park, we'd go to the beach, or we'd stop in a cafe. If there were any hitchhikers, we'd pick them up. Every time we stopped, we'd smoke a joint or give a joint away. We were all artists and we'd be drawing and getting stoned all day long."

Pioneering on the streets of San Francisco opened Swami up to an energy of exploration that would take him around the world. He experienced countless different religions, cultures, and spiritual perspectives but ultimately was drawn back to California. As cannabis became more and more viable as a legitimate business, Swami developed a relationship with Tim Blake as he was putting together the Emerald Cup. The Cup was developed as a platform to highlight the best of the best cannabis from growers adhering to practices that are in tune with the earth. As a founding judge for the cup, Swami found himself diving deep with other cannabis aficionados and also refining his joint-rolling abilities.

In the process of judging dozens and dozens of strains, Swami got insight into the power of joints as a clear and precise method to discern cannabis nuance. "For judging, you almost always have to smoke

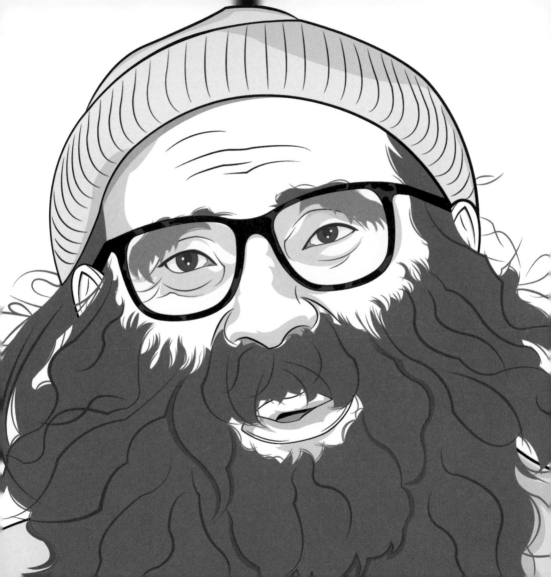

a joint," he says. "And one of the reasons for that is it's always clean. If you've got a bong or you've got a bowl, the first two hits might be clean, but every one after that isn't fresh." Swami explains, "There's maybe one hundred cannabinoids and who knows how many terpenes possible. As the joint burns, it guarantees that not only are you getting the cleanest smoke, but you are also getting the widest spectrum of compounds due to the gradual variation in temperature throughout the joint."

Swami's dog Tipu hops up next to him as he takes another puff on his joint. Overlooking the field of mature cannabis plants, he continues, "There's something very unique about the cannabis that's grown in California, especially in the Emerald Triangle. There is something specific to the climate, the geology, the geography, the water, and even the air that make this a very, very special place to grow." And it's through his commitment to culture and spirituality that Swami has been able to take all this knowledge and apply it on his farm. Engaging in only the most regenerative practices possible has put him on the forefront of cultivators who are growing plants in a truly sustainable way that benefits the earth, the plants themselves, and the people who smoke them.

"Up here in the mountains, there are still a few of us left. But, the hippies are dying off at a fairly fast clip these days," Swami says. He adds, "There is a certain sort of reverence for the relics, the OGs, you know, the few hippies who are still left. I've had several people tell me, 'You guys are heroes to us.'"

Thanks to decades of exploration and a commitment to earth-centric ideals, we have a perspective on the natural world around us that would be impossible without the vision of people like Swami and his peers. They are working to protect the land and create viable opportunities for farmers who aren't just focused on exploiting the plants and maximizing profits. This mission has been years in the making.

Taking the last few puffs on his joint as the Mendocino evening begins to creep in over the farm, Swami shares, "In those days in the hippie peak in San Francisco, we thought everybody was going to be turned on and we thought we were huge in numbers." He pauses, then concludes, "It turns out we were only a small group of people, but we've had a massive effect."

Swami Joint

The Swami joint is inspired by the culmination of years of regular smoking, traveling the world, and interacting with some of the most important cannabis connoisseurs alive today. Below are the instructions for how you can roll a Swami too.

Stash Box

Rizla papers (orange pack)
Roach clip
Silver cigarette case
Strike-anywhere matches

Instructions

1. Prepare your flower: Be sure to grind right before you smoke for maximum freshness. Grind it finely and consistently so you can pack as much as possible into the joint.

2. Prepare your paper: Refold the crease in your rolling paper so it has a slight taper toward the smoking end.

3. Fill the paper with as much flower as possible: The idea is to have as little extra paper as possible so the glue edge and the non-glue edge are lined up right next to each other.

4. Starting at the mouthpiece end, line up the paper, and lick the first third of the joint. Make sure you lick the back side of the glue: This will ensure you get the most glue remaining on the edge without licking it off.

Joint

9. Enjoy!

5. Hold your finger over the area you just licked for 5 or 10 seconds until it is dry. Repeat these steps for the middle third and end third of the joint.

7. Take a dry hit before lighting: This is a great way to savor the terpenes and flavor of the joint before you light it.

8. Carefully light the joint: It is almost like lighting a cigar. Light one edge, rotate it, light it again, and repeat this until the whole joint is well lit.

6. Get a tamper or something to help push more weed into the joint. Gradually fill up each side and push more and more down toward the mouthpiece end until the joint is very full.

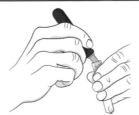

Clandestine Mission

The Godfather, the Packback, and the Secret Agent

If you like the idea of smoking one but you wanna keep things on the low, consider a more clandestine approach. Instead of rolling something up, you can simply empty out a cigarette or cigar and refill it with your favorite cannabis blend. It can take some patience, but when you are done you will have something that looks just like a commercial product. A cigar tube refilled with weed is called the Godfather and a cigarette tube refilled with weed (and sometimes with the filters replaced with paper tips) is called the Packback or Secret Agent. Now you just have to decide if you want your martini shaken or stirred!

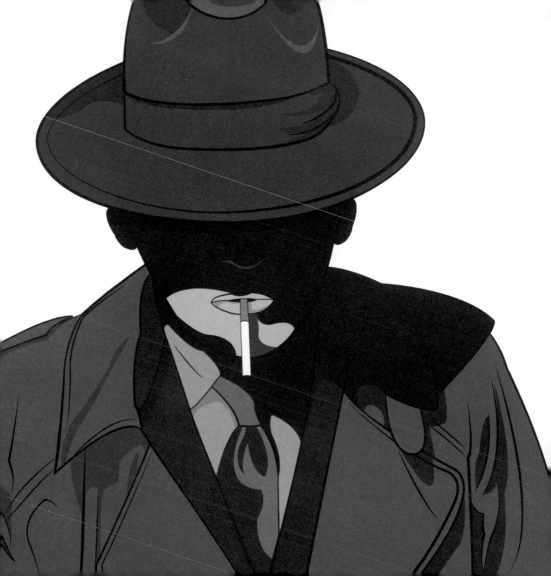

The Inside Out/Backward

The Inside Out is a simple twist on the classic roll that, because it has the smallest ratio of paper-to-smoking material, results in one of the cleanest ways to smoke a joint. It takes some practice and care, but it will change your rolling game forever. Plus, when you ignite the excess paper after you roll, it's kind of like doing a magic trick, and who doesn't like magic tricks?

Stash Box

1 king-size rolling paper
1 tip or filter
1 lighter

Instructions

1. Set your paper down with the glue side toward the table facing you.

2. Reverse the crease of the paper so it is now folded in the opposite direction of when it came out of the pack.

3. Place your filter tip in the paper.

4. Fill the paper with weed.

5. Very carefully roll with the glue side facing up, making sure there is no creasing.

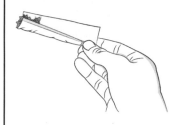

Joint

8. Gently make sure the glue has bonded with the paper and let it dry for 30 seconds.

6. Pull on the outside edge to keep the glue edge as flat as possible.

7. Find the glue line and moisten it through the layer of paper above it.

9. Carefully tear the extra paper, or if you are feeling more fabulous, you can light it on fire and watch the extra paper disappear.

Should I Smoke Another Joint?

1. Do you have to drive tonight?

A. No, I'm chillin'.
B. Yes, but I swear I got this.
C. Dude, where's my car?

2. How much do you have left in your stash?

A. An ounce of biodynamically grown NorCal outdoor.
B. Searching the ashtray for any half-smoked joints I can find.
C. A few grams left from this 4/20 event I went to last year.

3. How many pints of ice cream could you eat right now?

A. I'm vegan, thanks.
B. Cherry Garcia or Jerry Garcia—just can't make up my mind.
C. If you offered me an IV drip of Häagen-Dazs I wouldn't say no.

4. Did you drink anything?

A. Alkaline water, pH 9.1.
B. Just a couple shots (or five).
C. Cannabis-infused soda.

5. Do you have to accomplish anything tomorrow?

A. Discussing late capitalism with DMT elves.
B. My mom wants me to clean my room.
C. My boss wants to talk strategy for next quarter.

6. How comfortable is the couch you're on right now?

A. It's called a meditation cushion . . . look it up.
B. Can't quite tell; too many old pizza boxes between me and the cushions.
C. Total. Couchlock.

7. Is there an all-night drive-through nearby?

A. Already drank my last green juice for the day, thanks.
B. Gas station convenience stores are a totally legit source of nourishment.
C. Yo quiero Taco Bell.

8. When was the last time you put down your phone?

A. It's important to have boundaries with smartphone technology.
B. I can't wait to be one with the matrix.
C. Sooooo many cat videos.

9. What are you watching on TV?

A. Gregg Araki's *Smiley Face*.
B. Cable news on mute.
C. Shark Week binge.

10. Do you have to interact with any parents/authority figures/significant others?

A. I am accountable only to Jah.
B. My only relationship is with my PlayStation.
C. Yes, but I work at a dispensary.

11. What are you wearing right now?

A. Clothes are so oppressive, man.
B. Jeans and a T-shirt.
C. Sweatpants and slides.

If you answered mostly A's:

You are a motivated, enlightened individual with a clear perspective on the world around you. You have infinite potential. You should definitely smoke another joint.

If you answered mostly B's:

You have some growing up to do, but that's OK, we all start somewhere. You should definitely smoke another joint.

If you answered mostly C's:

You have trouble discerning between online horoscopes and real interpersonal advice. This may come back to haunt you later in life. You should definitely smoke another joint.

More Is Better

Bigger isn't always better, but when it comes to joints, blunts, and spliffs, sometimes it just is. If you feel comfortable with the basics of rolling standard joints and blunts, then going big is a great place to begin challenging yourself to uplevel your roll both functionally and visually. The basics here are like Lego™ bricks for smokers. Keep sticking papers and wrappers together, and you can go bigger and bigger. This is the cornerstone of all expansive rolls and opens the door to even the most decorative smokable sculptures.

L Paper Joint

First let's delve into making a two-paper joint called the L paper joint, so named because you are going to be sticking them together in the shape of—you guessed it—an *L*.

Stash Box

2 papers
Paper tip

Instructions

1. Lay one paper flat, then take the second paper and lick half of the glue strip.

2. Attach the two papers to make an L shape.

3. Now gently create a crease in the joint at an angle so it folds just below where the two papers meet for a 90-degree angle.

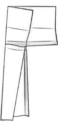

4. Fill the paper with herb and put in your paper filter.

Joint

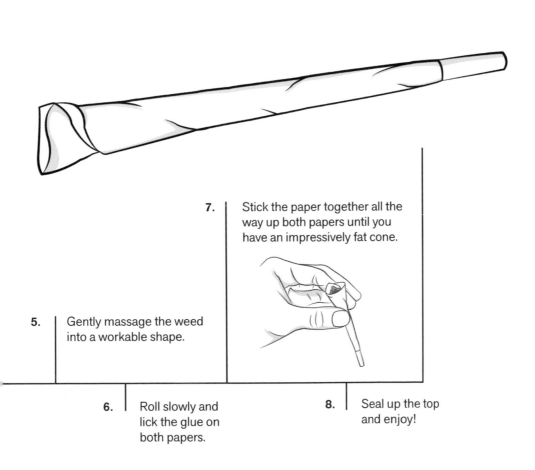

5. Gently massage the weed into a workable shape.

6. Roll slowly and lick the glue on both papers.

7. Stick the paper together all the way up both papers until you have an impressively fat cone.

8. Seal up the top and enjoy!

Mega/XXXL

If two papers aren't enough and you want to go for three, then rolling a fat three-paper joint is what you need in your life. Nicknames for this type of joint like the XXXL and the Mega are well deserved. Make sure you have at least 4 to 5 grams of weed to make these roll up right.

Stash Box

3 (1¼-size) rolling papers
4 to 5 tips

Instructions

1. Attach two papers together horizontally along the gum line to make an extra-wide paper.

2. Attach a third paper vertically on the side of the two papers that have already been attached. Make sure to note whether you intend to roll lefty or righty because the vertical paper makes more sense at the top of the joint.

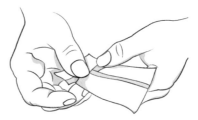

3. Roll a lot of paper tips. You'll need at least four or five tips rolled like you would for a normal cone joint.

4. Take all the tips you just rolled and wrap them together with one more piece of tip paper, making one big mega filter.

Joint

5. Add your weed to the big paper neatly. Start arranging it and get it ready to roll.

7. Carefully massage the herb into place while keeping the filters where they were and seal this bad boy up.

6. Place your large filter in the paper and make sure there isn't any weed between it and the paper.

8. Use a pen or other tool to push down the weed in the joint. Fold the extra paper down on the top and you are ready to go!

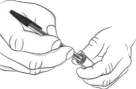

The Extendo

There's lots of ways to get more weed in a joint, but if you're bored of going fat, then you're ready to go extra long. It takes a steady hand to keep the balance of the Extendo while you're rolling it, but you will be rewarded once this lengthy joint comes to life.

Stash Box

2 king-size rolling papers
1 glue strip cut off of a king-size paper
Scissors
1 pen, screwdriver, or small rounded chopstick
1 tip or filter

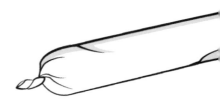

Instructions

1. Place your two papers glue side down on a table.

2. Take the glue strip you cut off the king-size paper, then cut it in half.

3. Moisten one glue strip and seal one side of the papers together, then repeat on the other side.

4. Place the papers now stuck together glue side up on your rolling tray.

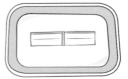

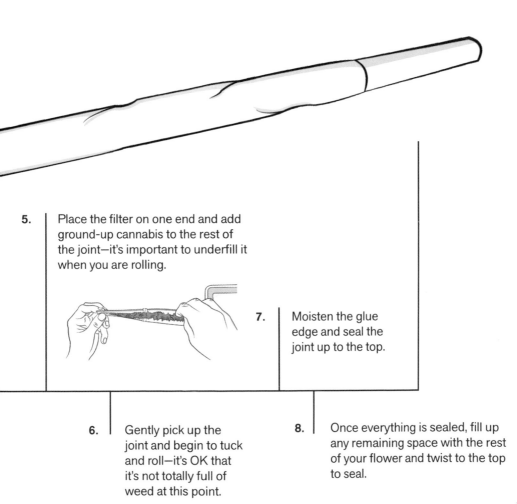

5. Place the filter on one end and add ground-up cannabis to the rest of the joint—it's important to underfill it when you are rolling.

6. Gently pick up the joint and begin to tuck and roll—it's OK that it's not totally full of weed at this point.

7. Moisten the glue edge and seal the joint up to the top.

8. Once everything is sealed, fill up any remaining space with the rest of your flower and twist to the top to seal.

Wiz Khalifa

Gettin' Paper by Rolling with Rolling Papers

From murdering mixtapes to crafting pop hits, Wiz Khalifa helped usher in a new chapter for hip hop that still reverberates today. The new chapter he helped birth isn't just about being unafraid of catchy pop hooks over perfectly crafted, propulsive beats—it's about artists being themselves, opening up about their fears and vulnerabilities, and not being afraid to confront their missteps (just as Khalifa did publicly after dropping a major label debut album that leaned so heavily into mainstream territory that his underground fans couldn't help but cringe).

Just as he is a pioneer in music, when it comes to rolling, Wiz is also a revolutionary. Defying decades of rap music's obsession with blunts of all kinds, Wiz burst on the scene with a commitment to rolling papers and joints that he credits with helping launch his career. Being a misfit isn't always as easy as it sounds, but Wiz's connection to classic, joint-smoking styles seems like a no brainer when viewed through the lens of what Wiz has brought with him to the world of music as a whole.

Look no further than the title to his debut album, *Rolling Papers,* for evidence of his fearless trailblazing and desire to show the world that any assumptions about him or the realm of rap in general are designed to be defied. When asked what inspired his rolling rebellion, he says, "I just found out joints were better and my life has been cleaner ever since."

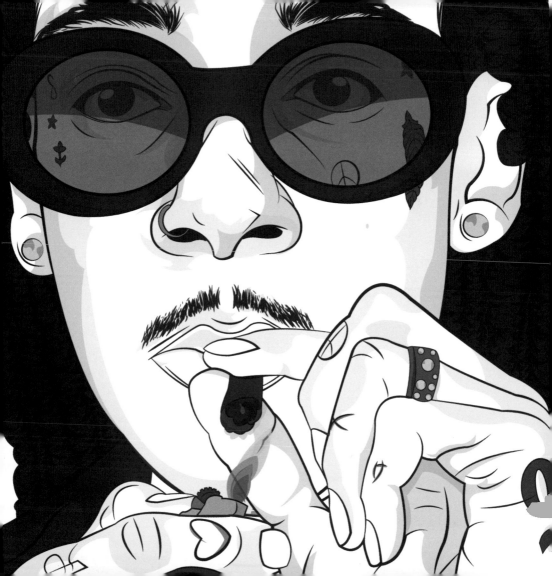

Roll Together

Why a Joint Might Be the Key to Relationship Success

Rolling a joint can do a lot of things, but did you know it can help you have a better relationship? Molly Peckler is a former matchmaker who uncovered the magic of cannabis in helping people with their love lives. The power of rolling joints, blunts, and spliffs (alongside other cannabis consumption methods) pushed her to pioneer a new approach to one-on-one matchmaking, date coaching, as well as larger-scale events focused on connecting through cannabis. Here she shares how a joint might be just what you need to overcome a variety of relatable relationship challenges.

Stress Relief

The world has gotten more stressful and many people suffer from anxiety. When you're anxious, you have a shorter temper and you are less empathetic. Being able to share a joint together is beneficial in reducing stress and helping you focus on the things that are most important.

Conflict Resolution

If you're having some sort of disagreement and you can't find that common ground, smoking together allows you to get out of your perspective. You can better listen to your partner and get over whatever issues or challenges are in the way, thus becoming more empathetic.

Sex

When the world gets crazy, sometimes sex is the first thing that falls off. But cannabis can help remind you of what's truly important. Sex is not everything in a relationship, but cannabis can help boost that desire or at least reduce some of the obstacles that get in the way of allowing you to enjoy sex and help you to stay connected both physically and emotionally.

Lightheartedness

When you and your partner can just laugh together, be silly and stupid, and not worry about being judged, it's incredibly powerful in creating a long-term bond. Laughter is always the best medicine, and cannabis is a great tool that allows you to see what's absurd and to laugh at the things that annoy you or even piss you off. You can see a much broader picture, and that can help make you feel better.

Great Sleep

Getting a good night's sleep is so important. If you're sleeping well, you are going to feel better, you're going to be happier, and you're going to be able to do whatever you need to do in your life. Sleep is one of the most powerful benefits of cannabis. I recommend smoking an indica-leaning strain to help you sleep through the night.

Ritual and Gratitude

When you utilize rolling and smoking as a ritual to slow down, set an intention, and think about what you want to achieve by consuming, it puts you into a different mindset. By taking time to clear your mind and enjoy a moment of peace, you can focus on the fact that you are so lucky to be with your partner and that you get to have this little escape, no matter how crazy the world around you is.

Roller's Worst Nightmare

May the Biggest Fail Win!

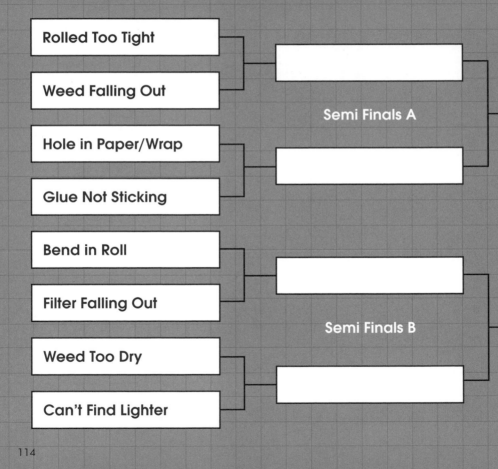

Rolled Too Tight

Weed Falling Out

Semi Finals A

Hole in Paper/Wrap

Glue Not Sticking

Bend in Roll

Filter Falling Out

Semi Finals B

Weed Too Dry

Can't Find Lighter

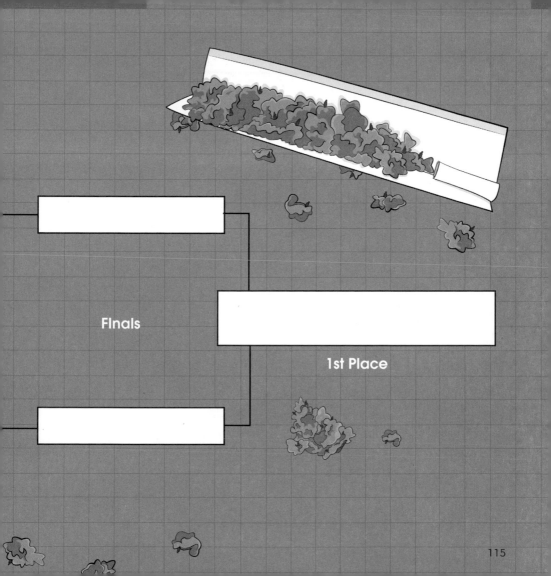

Finals

1st Place

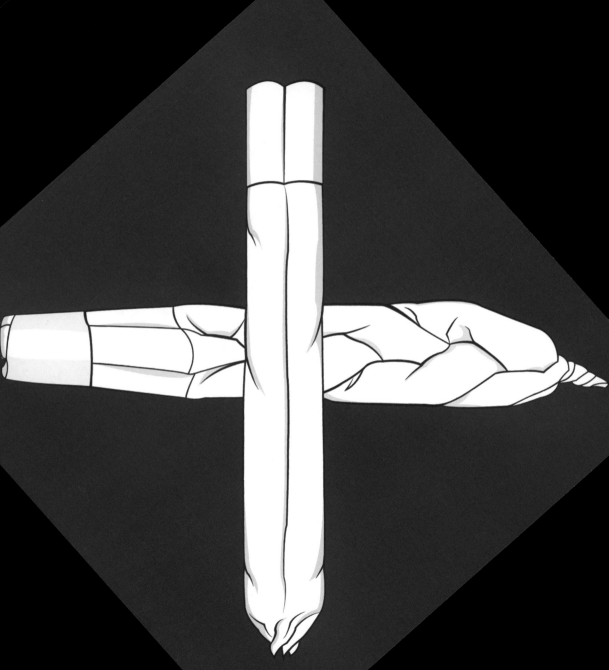

Adding Joints

If you've explored the possibilities of putting more papers together to create a bigger joint and are ready for another angle on how to step up your smoke, then you are ready to explore merging joints together. Two joints can form what is called the Double Barrel or Shotgun, and with three you can create what's sometimes called a Steamer. And if you're ready to get your swerve on, take three joints and put them together in the infamous Braid joint.

Shotgun

Because you are using extra paper in this method, it is recommended to roll them "inside out" or backward (see page 94). This will minimize the amount of paper you are smoking. Make sure the joints are small and identical in size because you will eventually need to fit both joints in a single piece of rolling paper.

Stash Box

3 (1¼-size) rolling papers

Instructions

1. Roll two Inside Out/Backward joints as small as possible and with the same diameter.

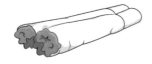

2. Take another paper and place the two joints you just rolled inside it.

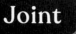

Joint

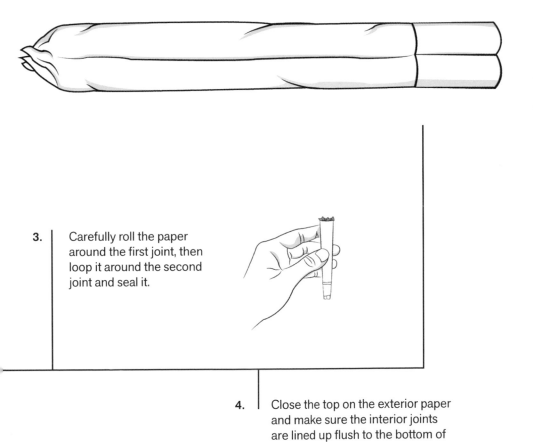

3. Carefully roll the paper around the first joint, then loop it around the second joint and seal it.

4. Close the top on the exterior paper and make sure the interior joints are lined up flush to the bottom of the paper.

Triple Braid

The Triple Braid is one of the funkiest-looking rolls you can pull off, but it's not without precedent. The "culebra" (which means "snake" in Spanish) is a type of triple-braided cigar that is thought to have originated in the Philippines in the 1800s before making its way to the United States several decades later. Anyway, enough cigar talk—roll up a few nice, long, thin joints and get ready to see what kind of snake you can make!

Stash Box

3 king-size rolling papers
3 paper tips
2 rolling paper gum strips

Instructions

1. | Roll three thin, long joints—be sure to under-fill them, as it will help with braiding them later.

2. | Gently twist the top of each joint to keep in the herb—you will untwist the joints shortly, so don't do it too tight.

3. | Align the three joints so the tips are in a triangular formation.

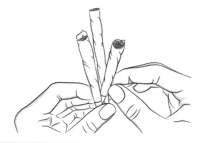

4. | Moisten your gum strips and wrap them around the three tips so they become one.

Joint

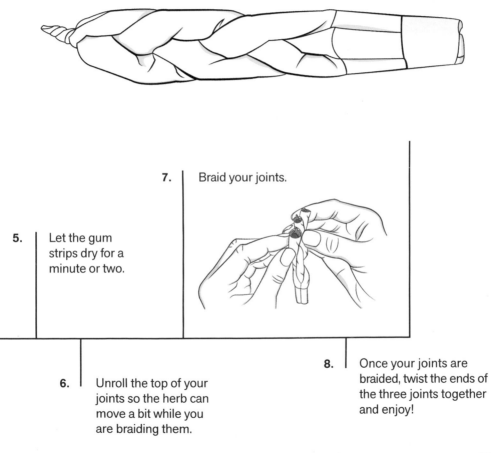

5. Let the gum strips dry for a minute or two.

6. Unroll the top of your joints so the herb can move a bit while you are braiding them.

7. Braid your joints.

8. Once your joints are braided, twist the ends of the three joints together and enjoy!

Roll Report:
United Kingdom

Burn enough zoots and you'll be chuffed to bits!

Fun Fact

In the late nineteenth century, medical cannabis was all the rage in England. Tinctures, pills, and syrups containing cannabis were frequently recommended by chemists in the know. You could even buy "Indian cigarettes" made by Grimault and Sons, which were essentially prerolled joints. Advertisements appeared in newspapers like *The Illustrated London News* and marketed the therapeutic spliffs as a cure for asthma, bronchitis, and "other affectations of the respiratory organs."

Dank Tourist Tip

Pay tribute to Dank of England legend Black the Ripper (RIP): Hit the London streets and light up everywhere you can. Some of the spots on the Ripper's list include the London Eye (where he conducted an infamous smoke sesh) and the residence and offices of the UK prime minister at 10 Downing Street (where he hung out with two ripe cannabis plants in his hands following a casual stroll through central London). If that all sounds a little too hot for your liking, make your way to Hyde Park on April 20 for their annual open-air smoke-out.

Key Vocab

Zoot	A joint
Backstrap	Inside-out joint
Chip	Tobacco that goes into a spliff
Fathead	Big-ended joint
Pinhead	Small joint
Warhead	Big, fat joint (over 8 grams)
L plate	L paper joint

More Powerful Joints, Blunts, and Spliffs

Concentrate on Concentrates

Sometimes you want a bigger joint, sometimes you want a smaller joint, but what if you want a more powerful joint? By adding concentrates of different kinds, either in your rolling material or on the outside of your joint, you can increase the percentage of THC and/or CBD, thus making whatever you are smoking a little (or a lot) punchier. This is also a realm where you can get more decorative with your joints, from using kief to dust the exterior of your roll to decorating it with a twirl of cannabis wax. You can even replace the entire exterior of your joint with a carefully hand-pressed piece of hash for a superior smoking experience.

Inside

When we feel mixed up inside it's generally not a pleasant experience. When our joints and blunts are mixed up on the inside, however, that's another story. From a dash of kief to adding bubble hash or wax, there are numerous ways to elevate your roll. You can even put "snakes in the grass" with extended threads of gooey hash or wax.

Outside

Some people say it's what's inside that counts. Most likely those people have never coated the outside of their joint or blunt with an otherworldly combination of dank cannabis concentrates. Adding a dusting of kief or a twist of wax can be the cherry on top of your roll. And if you're ready to go there, layer your exterior concentrates all together and you'll be getting intergalactic in no time.

Wayne Coyne

The Flaming Lips Front Man Knows the Art of the Deal

As much as the Flaming Lips are about art and music, I like that we have stuff. You know, there's a record you can buy. There's a concert you can go to. So I think for me, having THC and CBD products is just another way to say, look, I did this painting and I can talk about the painting as opposed to it always just being about me.

We made a gummy skull with a brain in it one time for a show that we were doing in a cemetery in Los Angeles. The brain was marijuana flavored. It didn't taste that good, but everybody that ate it mistakenly thought that it had a bunch of THC in it, but it didn't. I couldn't defeat this myth, so I'm forever known as the guy that made the skull that everybody believed had a THC gummy brain in it. We had a marijuana leaf on there and everything, though, so I can see why everybody thought that, of course.

My oldest brother is eight years older than me, so growing up, virtually everybody around me was smoking pot. Everybody's car that you got into and everybody's apartment you went to would just be constantly filled with pot. When I was sixteen I

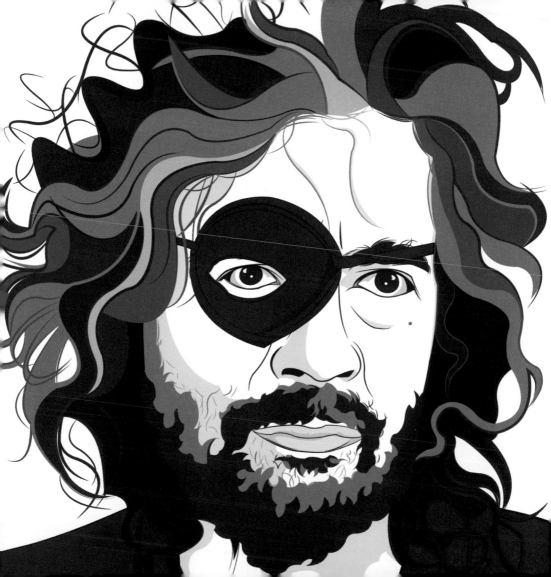

was working at a Long John Silver's restaurant but I got connected to this big-time pot dealer guy through my older brothers and all their friends, and I started selling weed out of my apartment.

I would end up driving in cars with my older brothers and their weed. It was the most potent weed ever and it would just be nonstop. Every time I went to roll a joint, I would attempt to do it and then someone who knew how to do it faster and better would just say, let me do that. So I never really got good at it.

I think around the time I was about to turn eighteen I just decided, "Look, this is OK. I've had a good run here. I'm going to get out before something bad happens." But it wasn't just because I turned eighteen. Like, I used to ride a motorcycle and I had the weed stuffed in the front of my coat and then a cop started following me. Of course with all that adrenaline I'm just thinking, "What am I going to do?" Luckily, nothing happened. But after that I decided I just don't want to mess with it, you know?

I was worrying about getting busted and going to jail, but really, I should have been more worried about these fucking weird old dudes that were coming to my apartment at four o'clock in the morning. I never considered that they could just walk in with a gun. I got very, very lucky. Naive is not even a good enough word for it, you know, just living in some dream left over from *Easy Rider* or something.

As told to Noah Rubin.

Cannabis Alchemy Pt. 2

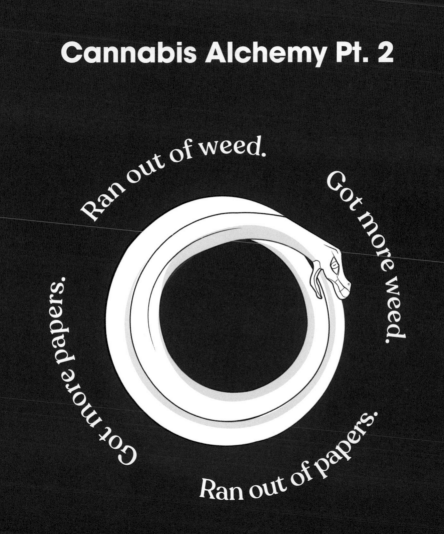

Ran out of weed.

Got more weed.

Ran out of papers.

Got more papers.

Roll Report:

ITALY

Hemp and hash history happened here.

Fun Fact

Some historians believe cannabis played a role in early Christian and Catholic religious rituals for hundreds of years. In Bible translations, some linguists argue that "cannabusum," which is described in the Bible as an ingredient in holy anointing oil, is a reference to cannabis. Now, that's how to get in touch with a higher power!

Dank Tourist Tip

Visit the Piazza Navona in Rome, grab a table, roll up a spliff, and people watch for the day. The Piazza features three notable fountains, including the Fontana del Moro. And no, contrary to what you might assume at first glance, the tritons in the fountain are not smoking huge joints.

Key Vocab

Cannone	Literally "a cannon": a cone-style joint
Bandiera	Literally "a flag": a common way to smoke in Italy "inside out"
Lungo	Literally "long": bigger is better, even in Italy
Primavera	Literally "spring": a spliff with cannabis flower alongside hash and tobacco

Match the Song with the Product or Rolling Style It Mentions

A.	Drake, "Hotline Bling" (2015)	**1.**	Fronto Leaf
B.	Chance the Rapper, "Smoke Break" (2015)	**2.**	RAW paper
C.	A Boogie wit da Hoodie, "Timeless" (2016)	**3.**	EZ Wider
D.	Megan Thee Stallion, "Go Crazy" (2020)	**4.**	White Owl
E.	Bad Bunny, "Yo Perreo Sola" (2020)	**5.**	Backwoods
F.	Wiz Khalifa, "Never Been" (2010)	**6.**	Phillies blunts

Answer Key: A:5, B:4, C:1, D:2, E:6, F:3

A.	UGK, "Swishas and Dosha" (2007)	**1.**	White Owl
B.	Nas, "Suspect" (1996)	**2.**	Phillies blunts
C.	Eazy-E, "No More ?'s" (1988)	**3.**	Swisher Sweets
D.	Wu-Tang Clan, "Wu-Tang: 7th Chamber Part II" (1993)	**4.**	Dutch Masters
E.	Gang Starr, "Take Two and Pass" (1992)	**5.**	Siamese blunts
F.	Redman, "Can't Wait" (1994)	**6.**	Zig-Zag

Answer Key: A:3, B:5, C:6, D:4, E:1, F:2

Laganja Estranja

Rolling a Joint Can Be Such a Drag

When I was becoming a drag queen, I was nervous to roll a joint, so I just smoked out of glass pieces. I didn't want to ask how to roll, because even though I wasn't Laganja in the beginning, I still felt like there was the stigma that came with weed smokers, like you just need to know how to do this. I explored cannabis a bit in high school, and I preferred a classic, grape-flavored blunt, a Swisher Sweet. The music that I grew up listening to in Texas has a kind of hood vibe, if you will, and they would talk about smoking Swishers, so that definitely perpetuated it among the younger crowd. Smoking Swishers was the rule and I followed. Backwoods are just a little strong for me.

Once I became Laganja Estranja, it was clear that I was going to have to be able to roll a joint. Everyone was always expecting me to do it and I had a reason to want to roll better. I was like, OK, I have to buckle down not only on my cannabis education, but being able to roll. I had three different people teach me three different techniques and I think I just kind of blended a little bit of all of them together. I roll with a crutch, and

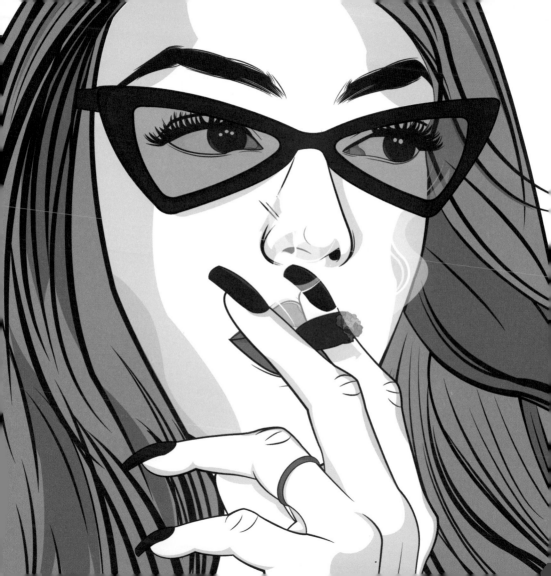

I roll with the sticky on the back side. The hardest part even to this day, especially with nails, is the tuck, lick, and roll.

I think joint rolling is an important thing to know how to do. You don't always have access to a piece, but you pretty much always have access to paper. I mean, I have used the Bible before, I'm not going to lie. It's a good technique to have because (a) of course, its thinness, its texture, the way Bible paper is similar to joint paper, and (b) there's always a Bible in a hotel. I do it without scripture or anything like that; I always use a front page or a back page. I wouldn't want to do the typed part because I think the ink would not be good.

I don't need to smoke with a celebrity to have the joint be special, but smoking with Miley Cyrus in her backyard and making art with her was such an unreal experience. Because I am the queen of cannabis, she was looking to me to bring her the right type of thing and I was able to give her the best of the best and smoke it with her. Her backyard is like a magical playland; she's got a big teepee and crazy signs. She was so real and vulnerable and revealed herself to me in those moments. But my biggest goal and dream is to smoke with Missy Elliott, that's who I really want to smoke with one day. She is an artist who wants to change the way we see things and wants to do it with pop culture. And I think as a drag queen, that's exactly what I'm trying to do.

As told to Noah Rubin.

Get Creative

Beyond Joints, Blunts, and Spliffs

Ever feel like your life is full of déjà vu? The same house, the same meals, the same shoes, the same routine . . . we've all been there. It happens with joint rolling too, and when that's the case, you've gotta spice up your next sesh. Grab a banana, an apple, or a pumpkin (or, if you're not feeling fruity, grab a store-bought multi-joint holder, a.k.a. a "trident") and jam as many joints as you want right inside. With the plume of multiple joints dancing away, there's no chance you can complain about being stuck in the same old dimension.

Films and TV Shows That Could Be About Weed, but Aren't

Just Roll with It (2017)

Just Roll with It is a family-friendly Disney Channel show where a live studio audience determines the fate of the show's cast. This usually means people getting splattered with paint, slimed with goo, and a variety of other icky-sticky nonsense. Spoiler alert: There is nothing icky or sticky that gets rolled up and smoked on this show.

Blunt Talk (2015)

Starring acclaimed Shakespearean actor Patrick Stewart, *Blunt Talk* sees Stewart play Walter Blunt, a television news host. Walter has a hard-partying dark side (mostly pills, powders, and booze) that he constantly needs to conceal from his often zany co-workers. On a scale of zero to ten blunts, this gets a zero.

The Man in the High Castle (2015)

Based on the Hugo Award–winning novel of the same name (penned by sci-fi visionary Philip K. Dick), *Man in the High Castle* imagines an alternate history in which the Nazis and the Japanese won World War II and split the United States in half. Though interdimensional excursions are a key part of the plot, sadly there is no one in this show who gets high in a castle.

Smoke Signals (1998)

Directed by Chris Eyre, *Smoke Signals* is considered one of the most authentic and compelling dramatic depictions of modern Native American reservation life ever. Coincidentally, there is also a Smoke Signals cannabis dispensary on the Algonquins of Pikwakanagan First Nation reserve lands in Ontario, Canada, that offers not only cannabis but also traditional medicines including a bear salve based on a 150-year-old recipe. Now, that's a win-win!

Gorillas in the Mist (1988)

This film offers a moving account of Dian Fossey's story of living with and studying endangered mountain gorillas. In one of her most memorable roles, Sigourney Weaver brings to life Fossey's battle to save one of our earth's most precious creatures. This leads to the obvious question: If you can teach a gorilla to do sign language, can you also teach it to roll a joint?

High Life (2018)

High Life is a chilling thriller about prisoners sent to conduct experiments in deep space with no chance of returning to earth. Starring Robert Pattinson and ringing up bonus points for André Benjamin's role, sadly no one smokes a joint in this movie. On the other hand, their spacecraft features an extraterrestrial garden that is definitely full of weed plants, so I'm guessing there must be a deleted scene somewhere on the editing room floor with a heady Pattinson/Benjamin intergalactic smoke sesh. Guess you'll have to wait for the director's cut.

L'roll Erotique

How a Joint Can Help You Step It Up in the Bedroom

A well-rolled joint is very sexy, but can it also be sexual? According to noted sex educator Ashley Manta, a.k.a. the CannaSexual, the answer is a confident yes. Ashley has committed herself to expanding her and her clients' sexual horizons by mindfully leveraging the power of cannabis. Not only is she the author of the pioneering sex book *The CBD Solution: Sex* but she has also been called "America's High Priestess of Pleasure" by *Sexual Health* Magazine. Her pioneering work with intimacy and cannabis even won her the honor of being the XBiz Awards' "Sexpert of the Year." Read on for some bedroom-friendly rolling insights from Ashley and prepare to never look at your joint the same way again.

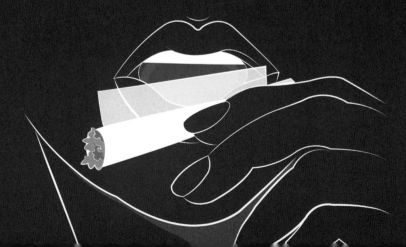

The Lick

The lick is a seductive technique. It is designed to entrance your lover with eye contact and deliberate slowed-down movement. It is reminiscent of your tongue on other parts of their body. You hold the joint in your fingers as you're ready to close it. You catch your partner's eye. You go so painfully slowly and you keep that eye contact as you're licking up the length of the joint. Every little bit of it, like a promise of what's to come.

The Fingers

The fingers are an essential tease. The dexterity that it takes to roll a joint or blunt is significant and there is a lot of skill involved. You get to show off how well you can manipulate your fingers toward a desired outcome. Your partner wants to know what those fingers are going to do to their body, so emphasizing how well you manipulate your fingers implies how well you can manipulate parts of your lover's body.

The Stroke

This is blatantly sexual and it's meant to be. During the rolling process, you are going to smooth out your joint or blunt by running it between your thumb and finger. You want your partner to think of what your hands could be doing on other body parts in your presence. The name of the game with all these techniques is slow. It's conscious and it's connected and it starts to give a hint of what's to come (pun intended).

The Presentation

There's something so beautiful about the rolling ritual, almost like when you go to a worship service and you know the protocols. There's lots of different ways that you can exchange the joint once it's rolled. It could be in your outstretched hand, it could be on a tray, or it could even be in between your lips where you just put it in a kiss and give it to them that way.

Blowing Smoke

I find it really hot when guys can do smoke tricks because the way that you form the smoke is by moving your tongue and arranging your lips in certain ways. This is suggestive of kissing and oral, like, "OK, you can do that with your mouth. I wonder what else you can do." The next level is to just open your lips slightly and let the smoke come out as it will. It forms these beautiful tendrils and is really cool to watch.

Shotgunning a Hit

This is an awesome way to connect with a partner, especially if you both smoke. If my partner has a bigger lung capacity than me, I appreciate them being the one that takes the first hit. Then they exhale and the receiving partner inhales, and then you can either pass it back and forth for a little bit or you can just both exhale and start kissing and have your tongues massaging each other and tasting the smoke together and connecting in that way.

Afterglow Indulgence

It's so lovely to have someone bring you a joint in bed after you've had an ecstatic experience with your partner. A lot of times you just kind of want to fall back and breathe it all in, but a joint or blunt can make you feel even better. So the act of service for your partner, to bring them something that they know is going to make them blissed out even more, is a beautiful way of showing care and affection in the relationship and in the interaction. As an upgrade, light the joint for them. I like to say that in my bed, no one lights their own joints.

Kinky Possibilities

A blanket caveat to all of this is that everything has to be happening consensually and that you have negotiated these terms prior, and that there's a safe word. So assuming that you've already established that both people are into it, there are power dynamics you can explore as part of a dominant/submissive relationship. You can have joints rolled and prepared for when your partner arrives and they are displayed and then you can light it for them. Or a command, like, "Go roll me a joint. I want to see you do it, and then I want you to bring it to me on your hands and knees," to create the experience of submission to your partner.

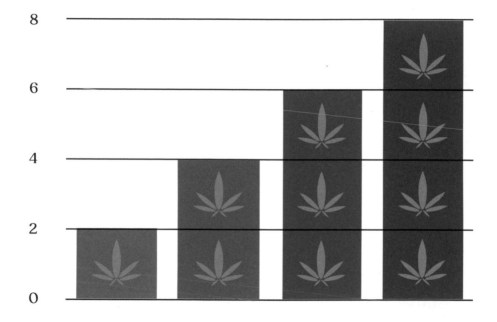

Does Weed Make You More Creative?

| Number of Joints Smoked | So many possiblities! | I could really use a snack right now. | (Yawns) I did wake up pretty early this morning... | How long have I been staring at my shoe? |

Dawn Doan, a.k.a. the Grasshoppa, Is the First Lady of Rolling

"What hasn't been done before is the ultimate with great rollers," says Dawn Doan, a.k.a. the Grasshoppa. "It has to be something new and it has to be something that touches people." Though far from a household name, Dawn is a pioneer of using rolling to make a human connection. She is the first ever female invited to join the National Joint League, a social media–centric competitive bracket–style rolling league that has made her, the league, and other luminaries from the crew highly sought-after artists and personalities known for making unimaginable rolling-paper magic.

"Every person in the community has their touch; we all have a different point of view," says Doan from her home on the Central Coast of California. "For me, what I give is new technology, new things you haven't seen, like my square joint, triangle joints, or even my Swiss [cheese] joint." The unprecedented creations that Dawn has shared with the world have brought her accolades not only among other top-tier rollers, but social media similarly can't help but take note.

Doan's story starts almost like a Hollywood movie–style immigrant tale. Displaced by the war in Vietnam, she spent time in refugee camps as a young child before moving to the United States and eventually settling in California with her family. The daughter of a nautical engineer, Doan and her family were able to embrace their immigrant journey with a proactive approach that sustained them comfortably. "We came to California and did farming," she reminisces. "You know, working the soil . . . I think that also segues into cannabis somehow."

Taking agricultural cues from her upbringing, Dawn became fascinated with growing cannabis. In spite of its dubious legal status in California at the time, Dawn was determined to take a stab at cultivating top-notch bud. "I flew to Canada to acquire seeds and I met Marc Emery, who was the prince of pot back then," Doan says. "I brought it back and grew it in a tent in the hills." This hands-on experience with cultivating the plant was also a seed for her interest in next-level creative rolling, stating plainly, "As a roller you have to have access to a lot of herb."

Her reputation for loving weed so much even earned her the nickname "the Grasshoppa." The nickname originated from her youth, when her family would joke about her aspirational love of kung fu, even though proper study of martial arts was reserved solely for her male siblings. The name later transformed into a perfect handle for Doan as she began exploring cannabis more deeply, especially because she was "always hopping around looking for weed."

Much like her nickname, her creative rolling instincts grew out of her family dynamic as well. She recalls holidays like Thanksgiving with her smoke-friendly relatives as moments for her to roll up something special. Taking cues from the back of the *High Times* magazines she was reading at the time to educate herself about growing, Dawn got insights into innovative rolling ideas that she would share with her family. "I would do a traditional cross joint or a braid joint or a big cannon," she says. But her ideas about what was possible soon changed.

"After seeing Tony's joint, I was like, OK, I can do more than this," says Dawn, referring to a Spider-Man figurine joint rolled by Tony Greenhand that she came across online. Tony is widely considered the world's top roller. He not only has a huge following online and a wide range of celebrity clientele ordering his custom sculptural rolls, but he has also branched out into entertainment. His show *Let's Roll* on the now-defunct platform Quibi was a glimpse into how high a roller can take their art. With Tony's posts in mind, plenty of plant material in hand, and just the right nickname for her pursuits, the Grasshoppa set out to do something beyond what she had previously thought possible.

"I've always loved cigar culture, and there's a cigar style called a box press cigar and it looks kind of square-ish," says Dawn. "For years I've wanted that as a joint, and after seeing Tony Greenhand's posts, I was like, OK, this is possible." And with possibility as her guiding mantra, Dawn set about rolling the box press–style joint, and needless to say, things went better than planned. Not only did she craft the unprecedented joint, but once she posted it online, the reaction was immediate. "Every major account reposted it," she says. "RAW [papers] asked me to be on their team and the National Joint League knocked on my door that same week. I was floored and honored."

Dawn's huge online splash was made even more significant as she simultaneously broke through a major glass ceiling. The cannabis industry is a very male-dominated space, but Dawn's belief in her ability to innovate helped her change the dynamic, at least within the rolling community. When asked about her feelings on being a pioneering female roller, she reflects, "I think for most females in the industry, it makes you want to prove yourself even more. I don't want to be the last girl getting picked on the field. I want to really come out and show." And to that she adds, "I love being an advocate for the females, that you can be in the space and do whatever you want."

And do whatever she wants, Dawn does, as she continues to set the bar high on all fronts. She's debuted numerous custom sculptural rolls that have lit the internet on fire. From a smokable WALL-E to a smokable Baby Yoda, she is an expert at taking pop culture cues and incorporating them in her smokable objects. In addition, she founded her own line of custom smokables called Luxe Rolls. She says, "I have really big visions of Luxe being Louis Vuitton or Murakami of this industry."

With such a high bar set for herself and an unwavering commitment to her craft (she reports that her smokable Baby Yoda took fifty hours to create), Dawn is no stranger to pushing herself. At the same time, she's looking to the future with more personal aspirations as well. "I want to roll for Lady Gaga," says Dawn when asked about her bucket list. "I know she smokes and I want to roll a figurine of her at a piano with one of her crazy outfits. She's such an art lover. I think she would just trip on it."

"I think for most females in the industry, it makes you want to prove yourself even more. I don't want to be the last girl getting picked on the field. I want to really come out and show. . . I love being an advocate for the females, that you can be in the space and do whatever you want."

What You Should Give Your Body When You're High AF

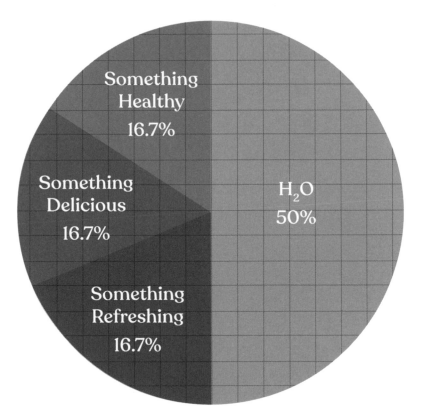

Something Healthy 16.7%

Something Delicious 16.7%

H_2O 50%

Something Refreshing 16.7%

What You Actually Give Your Body When You're High AF

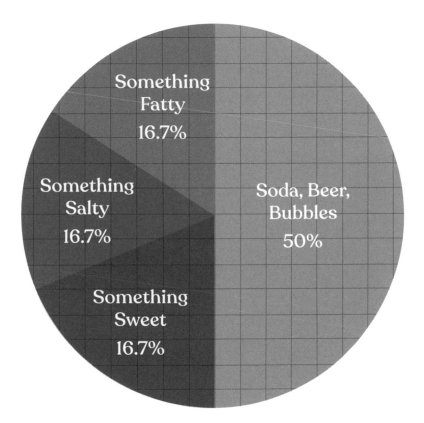

Something Fatty 16.7%

Something Salty 16.7%

Something Sweet 16.7%

Soda, Beer, Bubbles 50%

Popeye/Pipe

"Ceci n'est pas une pipe" ("This Is Not a Pipe") boldly states René Magritte in his iconic early twentieth-century surrealist painting *The Treachery of Images.* This work brings to our attention the material difference between a rendered image and reality itself. When you learn how to roll a sweet pipe joint, however, you can overcome this challenging paradox, as there's no question that you will be keeping it 100 percent real.

Stash Box

3 king-size rolling papers
1 paper tip
Lighter (BIC™, not Clipper™)
Scissors

Instructions

1. | Roll a nice, sturdy joint with a medium amount of taper toward the smoking end.

2. | Wrap a rolling paper around the lighter.

3. | Cut the gum strip off a piece of rolling paper and glue down the seam of the paper that is wrapped around the lighter.

4. | With your scissors, cut the end of the joint you rolled at a 45-degree angle, exposing the inside of the joint.

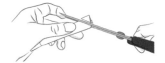

Joint

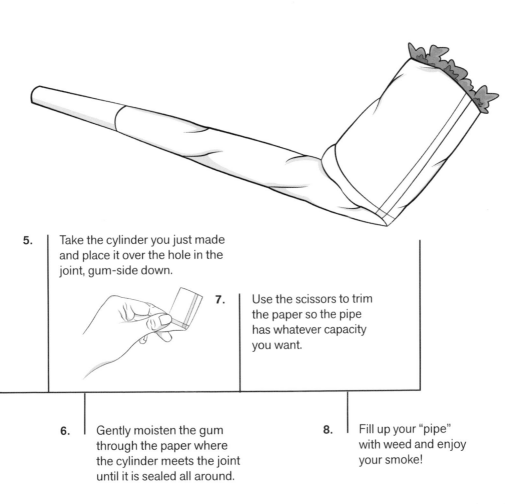

5. Take the cylinder you just made and place it over the hole in the joint, gum-side down.

7. Use the scissors to trim the paper so the pipe has whatever capacity you want.

6. Gently moisten the gum through the paper where the cylinder meets the joint until it is sealed all around.

8. Fill up your "pipe" with weed and enjoy your smoke!

The Cross

Sometimes you come to a crossroads in your life and you have to make the important decision of which path you will travel. With a cross joint, it's an opportunity to travel down the road of ever-more-interesting approaches to rolling up your favorite herb. Once you open the door to previously unknown rolling journeys, the sky will truly become the limit.

Stash Box

1 king-size rolling paper
1 tip or filter
1 (1¼-size) rolling paper
1 safety pin or paper clip
Scissors
1 pen, screwdriver, or small rounded chopstick
4 extra rolling papers for glue strips

Instructions

1. | Roll a big, fat joint with a tip or filter at the end.

4. | Cut a hole in the side of the big joint and then use the small, rounded chopstick to clear a hole all the way through the fat joint.

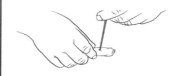

2. | Roll a small joint.

3. | Poke several little holes around the middle of the small joint.

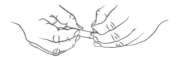

Joint

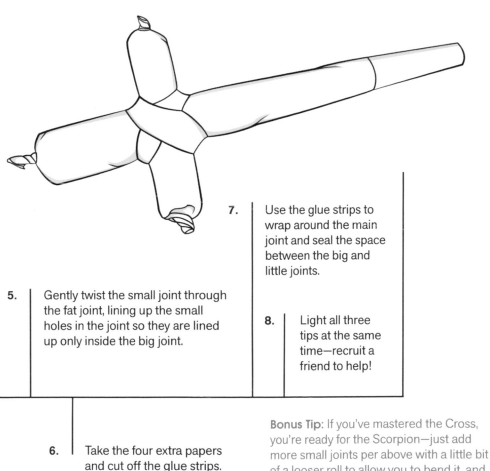

7. Use the glue strips to wrap around the main joint and seal the space between the big and little joints.

5. Gently twist the small joint through the fat joint, lining up the small holes in the joint so they are lined up only inside the big joint.

8. Light all three tips at the same time—recruit a friend to help!

6. Take the four extra papers and cut off the glue strips.

Bonus Tip: If you've mastered the Cross, you're ready for the Scorpion—just add more small joints per above with a little bit of a looser roll to allow you to bend it, and you will have a fully smokable sculpture!

The Tulip

Tulips are an inspiring flower. However, as the Dutch learned in the early 1600s, tulip inspiration can go too far. During Dutch tulipmania, people spent outlandish sums of money on trendy tulip bulbs. Speculative bulb bubbles aside, rolling up a sweet tulip joint and reflecting on the importance of intrinsic value versus collective hype is a worthy pursuit. But enough with the flowery language and on to this deep, dank roll!

Stash Box

3 king-size rolling papers
1 large piece of rolling tip-style paper (approximately the same length and width as the king-size paper)
1 piece of string

Instructions

1. Take two pieces of king-size paper and attach them to create an extra-wide paper.

2. Fold one end up toward the glue edge, creating a triangle.

3. Moisten the glue edge and seal it, creating a small cone.

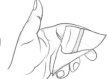

4. Fill the cone with well-ground flower.

Joint

5. Take a piece of tip-style paper and roll it. It should resemble an extra-long paper tip.

6. Wrap the tip-style paper with the third piece of king-size paper and seal it (this will be the tulip's "stem").

7. Take your stem and place it in the middle of your cone.

8. Tighten the paper around the stem by twisting and crumpling it around the stem.

9. Secure the paper over the stem with the small piece of string and get ready to enjoy your tulip!

Bonus Tip: Multiple tulips together make a beautiful bouquet. It's a perfect gift if your lover loves a classy roll.

Important Things to Remember

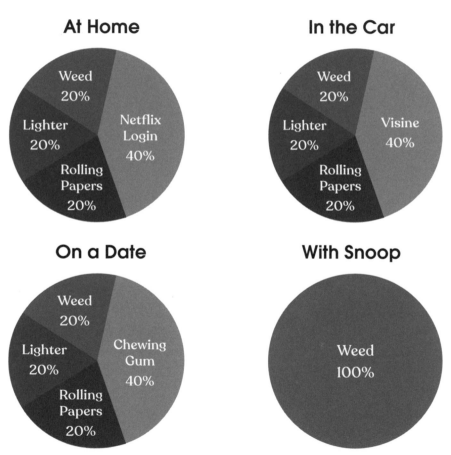

At Home

- Weed 20%
- Lighter 20%
- Netflix Login 40%
- Rolling Papers 20%

In the Car

- Weed 20%
- Lighter 20%
- Visine 40%
- Rolling Papers 20%

On a Date

- Weed 20%
- Lighter 20%
- Chewing Gum 40%
- Rolling Papers 20%

With Snoop

- Weed 100%

The End.

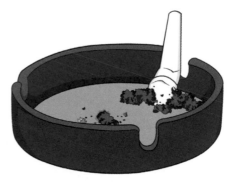

ACKNOWLEDGMENTS

First and foremost, I would like to give love and thanks to all the people who shared their time, knowledge, connections, and weed with me. You were essential in making this book possible. To anyone I forget to name below, apologies in advance, the weed is good and there's a lot of it.

Thanks to Tasia Prince for bringing this book to life with her amazing illustrations.

Thanks to my friends around the globe who brought their worldly perspectives on rolling that I feel are such an important ingredient in this book: Gamal Helmy, Luca Andrea Collins, Canni Danni, and Reece Yaboh.

Thanks to the other advocates and dot connectors who were essential in helping me tell a bigger and better story than I ever thought possible: Will Dzombak, Nicolas Morganstern, Kimberly Witherspoon, Paul Sommerstein, Jonathan Lyons, Josiah Adams, Kevin Muise, Evan Eneman, Michael Scherr, Karan Wadhera, Zach Fernandez, and Aaron Fogelson.

Thanks to the friends and family who have supported me on this journey, given me feedback, and helped me see how far I could take these ideas: my father, Lanny Rubin, my mother, Elizabeth Strasser, my brother, Ezra, as well as Sacha Jenkins, Julia Mayer, Chris Coady, Boshra AlSaadi, Madeleine von Froomer, Zach Sokol, Iris Alonzo, Jay Escobara, KP Lawless, Cory Shaw, Zainne Saleh, and Nikki Lastreto (plus Swami and Tipu too!).

Extra special thanks to Kendra Adler: Your emotional, creative, and spiritual support has been indispensable to me…and your enthusiasm never ceases to inspire.

Also, the most major thanks to the team at Chronicle Books past and present whom I have relied on in so many ways. On this project especially: Rebecca Hunt and Maggie Edelman, and since day one: Camaren Subhiyah, Sarah Billingsley, Lizzie Vaughan, Christine Carswell, Christina Loff, and Christina Amini.

This book is dedicated to all of the people behind bars who are unjustly serving time due to the racist and exploitive war on drugs. May your suffering soon end.

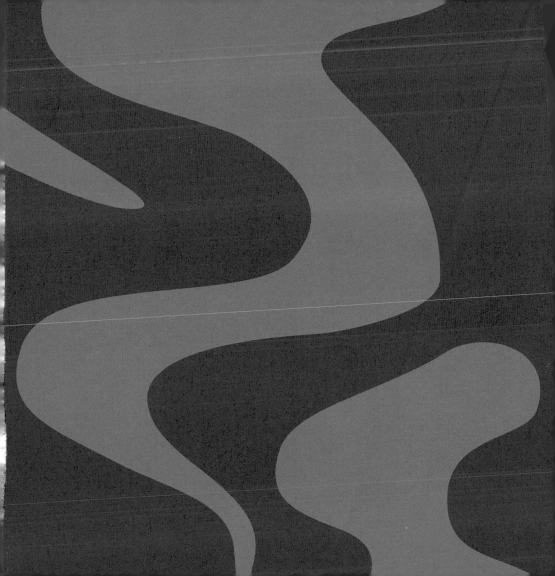

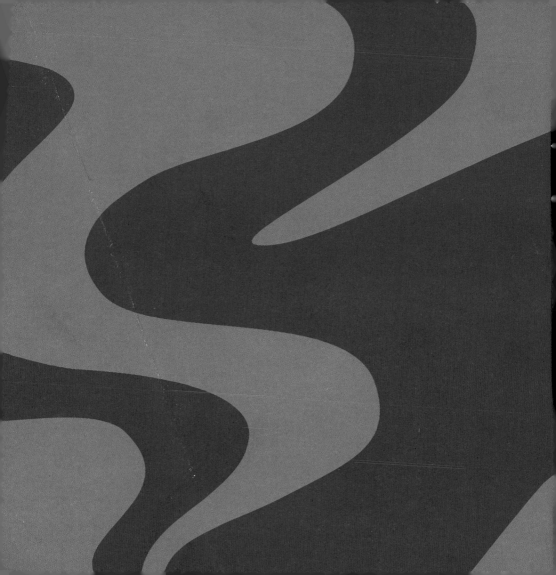